ALSO BY SHERWIN B. NULAND

How We Die

How We Live

Doctors: The Biography of Medicine

The Mysteries Within

Leonardo da Vinci

Lost in America

The Doctors' Plague

Maimonides

THE ART OF AGING

THE
ART
OF
AGING

A Doctor's Prescription for Well-Being

SHERWIN B. NULAND

RANDOM HOUSE / NEW YORK

Published in the United States by Random House, an imprint of The Random
House Publishing Group, a division of Random House, Inc., New York.

RANDOM HOUSE and colophon are registered trademarks of Random House, Inc.

Portions of Chapter 7 were originally published in different form as
"Do You Want to Live Forever?" in *Technology Review*, 108 (2) 36–45,
February 2005; portions of Chapter 8 were originally published in different form
as "How to Grow Old: A Physician's Prescription" in *Acumen: Journal of Sciences*,
1 (11) 48–57, August/September 2003 and "Pumping Iron" in *The American
Scholar*, the Journal of the Phi Beta Kappa Society, 68 (3) 121–124, Summer 1999.

Grateful acknowledgment is made to the following for permission
to reprint previously published material:

MIRIAM GABLER: Essay entitled "Long Overdue" by Miriam Gabler,
copyright © 2003 by Miriam Gabler. First published in *Ozarks Senior Living*,
Springfield, MO. Reprinted by permission.

RANDOM HOUSE, INC.: "Grace" from *Absolute Trust in the Goodness of the Earth:
New Poems* by Alice Walker, copyright © 2002 by Alice Walker. Reprinted by
permission of Random House, Inc.

SIMON & SCHUSTER ADULT PUBLISHING GROUP: Excerpts from
As I Am: An Autobiography by Patricia Neal, copyright © 1988 by Patricia Neal.
Reprinted by permission of Simon & Schuster Adult Publishing Group.

ISBN 978-1-4000-6477-9

LIBRARY OF CONGRESS CATALOGING-IN-PUBLICATION DATA
Nuland, Sherwin B.
The art of aging: a doctor's prescription for well-being / by Sherwin B. Nuland
p. cm.
ISBN-13: 978-1-4000-6477-9
1. Older people.   2. Aging.   3. Older people—Conduct of life.   I. Title.
HQ1061.N92 2007   305.26—dc22   2006049267

Printed in the United States of America on acid-free paper

www.atrandom.com

2 4 6 8 9 7 5 3 1

FIRST EDITION

Book design by Casey Hampton

TO MANNY PAPPER
wisdom, equanimity, caritas

Father Time is not always a hard parent, and, though he tarries for none of his children, often lays his hand lightly upon those who have used him well.

—Charles Dickens, *Barnaby Rudge*, 1841

CONTENTS

THE ART OF AGING

ONE

AN INCIDENT
IN THE SUBWAY

About five years ago, I had a brief experience that since then has helped me to tell the difference between nurturing a sense of vibrant good health and nurturing the delusion of being still young. Put somewhat differently, I learned that a man of advanced years who has never felt himself hemmed in by chronology should nevertheless not allow himself to forget his chronology entirely.

The event took place late on a September afternoon when I, along with my wife and younger daughter, had just entered a New York subway car at the Times Square station. Pushed forward by the advancing throng of rush hour passengers, we were crammed together single file, with nineteen-year-old Molly in the middle and me packed in behind her. Between my back and the doors stood someone whom my peripheral vision had recognized only as a tall, broad-shouldered man, perhaps in his late thirties. No sooner had the train gotten under way than the fellow's bare right arm reached around past me, its hand extending forward in an obvious attempt to make contact with Molly's buttocks. As taken aback as I was by the man's brazenness, I did have the presence of mind to do what any father might: I pressed my body rearward just firmly enough to push him up against the car's door, putting Molly beyond the reach of his outstretched fingers. As though by some form of unspoken New York agreement, both he and I acted as though nothing had happened, and the train continued on its clattering way over the subterranean tracks.

But I was wrong to think that the episode was over. Scarcely half a minute had passed before I became aware of a barely perceptible creeping thing, surreptitiously entering the right-hand pocket of my khaki trousers. Any thought that imagination was playing tricks on me was dispelled a moment later when I was able to feel an unmistakable sensation through the fabric, of fingertips moving around inside the empty pocket.

In the flashing eyeblink of time that followed, it never occurred to me that I should consider the consequences of what I instantaneously decided must be done. In fact, "decided" is hardly the word—my next actions were virtually automatic. I plunged my hand into the pocket, transversely surrounded the bony knuckles of a palm wider than my own, and squeezed down with every bit of force I could muster. Aware that I was gritting my teeth with the effort, I did not let go until I felt more than heard the sickening sensation of bone grating on bone and then something giving way under the straining pressure of my encircling fingers. A baritone roar of pain brought

me back to my seventy-one-year-old self, and made me realize that I had gone too far.

What had I let myself in for? Would not the simple act of
removing the intruding extremity have sufficed? Or perhaps I
should have done nothing—the pocket was, after all, as
empty as it always is when I anticipate being in a crowded,
chancy place. Made overconfident by hundreds of hours
spent pumping iron in a local gym, I had succumbed to an unthinking impulse dictating that I crush the felonious hand. As
the first flush of instinct faded, I all at once became certain
that my victim's revenge would now swiftly follow. Alarmed
by that thought, I relaxed my grip and felt the mauled ap-
pendage whip out of my pocket.

But who could have predicted that the response would
take the form that it did? With his torso still pressed up between my back and the train's doors, my antagonist inexplic-
ably shouted out a garbled accusation for all to hear, about
my having ". . . TRIED TO STEAL MY BAG!" Being certain
that I had misheard and anticipating a powerful assault, I
awkwardly turned my body around in those compressed
quarters, in order to confront the expected assault as effectively as my acute attack of nervous remorse might allow.
Having managed that, I found myself looking up into the an-
guished but nevertheless infuriated face of a thuggish-looking
unshaven tough three inches taller than I, and quite a bit
broader. I noted with some relief that the injured right hand
hung limply alongside his thick-chested body. Tucked up into
his left armpit was a bulging deep-green plastic portfolio, its
top barely held closed by a tightly stretched zipper. This, no
doubt, was the pouch in which was held the loot of a day's
pocket pilfering.

Seeing the flaccid, useless hand dangling from the muscular but now inactivated forearm momentarily revived my unthinking and foolhardy courage. Looking directly into the bloodshot eyes glowering at me (and now able to smell liquor on the thick breath blowing down into my face), I roared back as though I were Samson, "YOU HAD YOUR HAND IN MY POCKET!" Something stopped me before I added "you son of a bitch," which was a lucky thing because as soon as the first words were out of my mouth, I regretted them. Fearful once more, I prepared for the violent response that would surely follow.

But the fates were with me: Just at that moment, the train pulled into the next station and my foeman charged out through the doors as they slid open, clumping off toward an exit staircase as fast as he could, until his forward motion was slowed by a bunched-up throng of passengers tumbling out of the next car. He was swallowed up among them until only the top of his bobbing head could be seen. In a moment he was gone, leaving me standing there—thinking of how close I had come to my own annihilation.

I turned toward Molly and my wife, who later told me that my face was pale and bloodless. I felt as though rescued from certain death by a last-second reprieve. My hands were shaking and my knees seemed just a bit uncertain about whether they intended to continue holding me up. It was several minutes and another station's traveling before they steadied themselves. But everything finally stabilized and I was then faced with the embarrassment of having to withstand the two women's justifiably withering comments about how foolish I had been. During the short period of Sturm und Drang, they later told me, not a single person in that overcrowded subway car had so much as glanced in my direction or otherwise acknowledged that anything unusual was taking place.

I present this story as an example of a conflict within myself, a conflict that I suspect exists in the minds of many men and women beyond the age of perhaps their middle fifties. On the one hand, we recognize that age is ever increasing its effects on us and now requires not only acceptance but a gradually changing way of thinking about ourselves and the years to come; on the other, some narcissistic genie within us cannot give up clinging to bits of the fantasy that we can still call on vast wellsprings of that selfsame undiminished youth to whose ebbing our better selves are trying to become reconciled.

The same formula that enhances our later years—continued mental stimulation, strenuous physical exercise, and unlessened engagement in life's challenges and rewards—sometimes fosters an unrealistic confidence that the vitality thus maintained means that we are virtually the same as we were decades earlier, even in appearance, ready to challenge youth in its own arenas. In outbursts of denial and bad judgment that are virtually instinctual, we at such times discard an equanimity that has taken years to develop, and indulge ourselves in behavior foolhardy and foolish, as though using it as an amulet to stave off the very process to which we have so successfully been accommodating by consciously sustaining our bodies and minds.

The tension between the two is very likely stronger in the case of men, but nonetheless common in women as well, though manifesting itself in somewhat different forms. This rivalry within ourselves reflects a rivalry with youth, and it serves neither youth nor age at all well. Self-images from an earlier time are not easy to give up, even when giving them up is in our own best interest. Those whose calling is to work with an older population know that the ability to adapt, to learn and then accept one's limitations, is a determinant of what the professional literature of geriatrics calls "successful aging."

Adapting is not mere reconciling. Adapting brings with it the opportunity for far greater benisons and for brightening the later decades with a light not yet visible to the young. Even the word itself is insufficiently specific to convey what is required. In the subtle but nevertheless enormously significant shades of meaning that characterize the English language, "attune" may, in fact, better describe the process than "adapt": "attune," in the sense of being newly receptive to signals welcome and unwelcome, and to a variety of experiences not previously within range, while achieving a kind of harmony with the real circumstances of our lives.

This book is about attuning to the passage of years, and finding a new receptiveness to the possibilities that may present themselves in times yet to come—possibilities conveyed in wavelengths perceptible only to those no longer young.

And the book is also about traps for the unwary, into which all of us fall from time to time and from which we must teach ourselves to emerge with a refreshed sense of purpose. The very word—"attune"—sounds like another word to which it has a not coincidental connection: "atone," originally a contraction of "at one," meaning "to be in harmony," most cogently with oneself. To become attuned to an evolving perspective on a life is to be at one with the reality of the present and of the future years. Achieving such attunement can bring a form of serenity previously unknown, and perhaps unsuspected. The process begins with an acknowledgment that the evening of life is approaching. But with that approach come foreseeable possibilities. We have only to take advantage of all that those coming decades have in their power to offer. It is incumbent on each of us to cultivate his or her own wisdom.

So gradual a progression is the onset of our aging that we one day find it to be fully upon us. In its own unhurried way, age soundlessly and with persistence treads ever closer behind us on slippered feet, catches up, and finally blends itself into us—all while we are still denying its nearness. It enters at last into the depths of one's being, not only to occupy them but to become their very essence. In time, we not only acknowledge aging's presence within us, but come to know it as well as we knew—and still covet—the exuberant youth that once dwelt there. And then, finally, we try to reconcile ourselves to the inescapable certainty that we are now included among the elderly.

Realizing how much of our dreams we must concede to that unalterable truth, we should not only watch our horizons come closer but allow them to do precisely that. If we are wise, we draw them in until their limits can be seen; we confine them to the possible. And so, the coming closer can be good, if by means of that closeness—that limiting of expectations—we begin to see those vistas more clearly, more realistically, and as more finite than ever before. For aging can be the gift that establishes the boundaries of our lives, which previously knew far fewer confines and brooked far fewer restrictions.

Everything within those boundaries becomes thus more precious than it was before: love, learning, family, work, health, and even the lessened time itself. We cherish them more, as the urgency increases to use them well. Many are the uses of the newly recognized limits. Among their advantages is that our welcoming acceptance of them adds to the value, adds to our appreciation, adds to our ability to savor—adds to every pleasure that falls within them. The good is easier now to see; it is closer to the touch and the taking, if we are only willing to look truthfully at it there and gather it up from amid the cares that may surround it. There is much to savor during this time, magnified and given more meaning and intensity by the very finitude within which it is granted to us.

Aging has the power to concentrate not only our minds but our energies, too, because it tells us that all is no longer possible, and the richness must be more fully extracted from the lessened but nevertheless still-abundant store that remains. From here on, we must play only to our strengths. Some of the more meaningful of those strengths may be not at all less than they once were. The later decades of a life become the time for our capabilities to find an unscattered focus, and in this way increase the force of their concentrated worth.

Even as age licks our joints and lessens our acuities, it brings with it the promise that there can in fact be something more, something good, if we are but willing to reach out and take hold of it. It is in the willingness and the will that the secret lies, not the secret to lengthening a life but to rewarding it for having been well used. For aging is an art. The years between its first intimations and the time of the ultimate letting go of all earthly things can—if the readiness and resolve are there—be the real harvest of our lives.

It is the purpose of this book to tell of human aging and its rewards—and also of its discontents. And the book has as its purpose as well to tell of how best to prepare for the changes that inevitably demand accommodation, demand a shift in focus, and demand a realistic assessment of goals and directions, which may be new or may be a rearrangement of the trajectory of a lifetime. We do this at every stage of life without noticing the new pattern to which we are becoming attuned, whether it be in adolescence, the twenties, or middle age. Though the changes may be more obvious as we approach our sixties and seventies, they are, in fact, only a continuation of everything that has come before. For becoming what is known as elderly is simply entering another developmental phase of life. Like all others, it has its bodily changes, its deep concerns, and its good reasons for hope and optimism. In other words, it has its gains and it has its losses. The key word here is "developmental." Unlike most other animals, the human species lives long beyond its reproductive years, and continues to develop during its entire time of existence. We know this to be true of our middle age, a period of life that we consider a gift. We should recognize and also consider as a gift that we continue to develop in those decades that follow middle age. Living longer allows us to continue the process of our development.

Each of us concedes the onset of aging at our own moment; every man and woman acknowledges its beginnings and, finally, its fullness at a different time and for different reasons. As distinctive individuals, we experience it through our own bodies and the events of our own journeys. At fifty-two, Robert Browning already knew enough of such things to understand that their process was the accompaniment of their recompense. Aware that he had already exceeded the life expectancy of his era but not knowing that he would be granted twenty-seven remaining years in which to follow his own counsel, he famously had Rabbi Ben Ezra tell his congregation to:

> Grow old along with me!
> The best is yet to be,
> The last of life, for which the first was made:

And advised them that age is the time to:

> . . . take and use thy work:
> Amend what flaws may lurk,

But perhaps most important of all:

> Look not thou down but up!

It would hardly be realistic to paint the process of aging with a brush that Pollyanna or Pangloss might have used. The benisons of advancing age come with its burdens, and in some ways are the result of them. The one cannot exist in the absence of the other, and we should not hesitate to acknowledge the losses that accompany the gains. Nothing is accomplished by soft-pedaling the physical and emotional realities of aging. Were I to close my own and the reader's mind to all that is there, I would be unable to accomplish my aim, which is to tell of how to prepare for and face those realities, not only with equanimity but with the means to impede or lessen the most baleful effects of aging's onslaught—and, in fact, to use these losses when using them is a means to accomplishing the goals we may set for ourselves.

I have spent a career of almost forty years in a branch of surgery in which by far the greatest and most frequent challenges occur in treating men and women in late middle age and beyond. Their response to physical, emotional, and spiritual crises has been the stuff of my daily observations, and I have come to know both the frailty and the strength, the vulnerability and the resilience, that is theirs. They have been my patients, my friends, and my teachers, even when I was a young physician. Most recently, they have been me. In writing this book, I hope to return some of the gifts of knowledge and understanding that these men and women have given me over many years, and to share with others what I have learned. In all of this, my theme is Browning's "Grow old along with me!"—exclamation mark and all—for I am taking the journey even while I describe it, and I intend that my readers and I will continue to look up, while never forgetting to look down now and then.

But why look down? After all, the poet admonishes us against it, and dozens of self-help volumes tell us of the glories of that perpetual image of youth that can be ours if we but follow some simple directions. But all manner of promissory notes on an anti-aging future tend to ignore the obvious fact that, optimism or no optimism, steps are most sure when watchfully taken. We must see where our feet are truly placed and where they can still take us; we must not only gaze upward at the beckoning promise of retained intellectual and physical vigor, but we must be sensible and cautious, with a realization: What the unextinguished youthful spirit wills or imagines is not always what the aging flesh allows. The admonition "Act your age" has been applied to every stage of life, but it is in the older decades that it takes on a meaning beyond the mere avoidance of making a fool of oneself. These are lessons we must learn as the years pass. Prudent reality is a secret of vibrant survival, to temper the whiff of yesterday that sometimes urges us toward yearnings for what is beyond the possible. We must teach ourselves to recognize residual instinct that was useful at an earlier time of life, and rein it in with the bridle of good sense. The aim is to tell the difference between fact and fantasy; the aim is to guide oneself toward fulfillment of the reasonable.

There is a tyranny in decades; life should not be measured in ten-year packages. Moving on from one to the next is fraught with artificial implications. Whether the number of the supposed turning point is thirty or seventy, it comes with the expectation that we will thereafter be different from how we were before—that we are all at once somehow altered. We treat those seemingly defining moments in what is actually a process of imperceptible transition as though they bear a significance they do not in fact have—as though they are catalysts for an abrupt physical and mental transformation, when they are in reality no such thing. The truth is that the day of transition from one ten-year interval to another is merely a milestone, but we use it instead as a signal that somehow something has changed, or should change. A new set of expectations is inflicted on us—and we inflict it on ourselves—as we leave one cohort and enter another.

Our bodies, for example, do not know the difference. From the viewpoint of their biology, the final morning of fifty-nine is very much like the first morning of sixty. And yet, our minds have already set themselves to a new rhythm. We think we are older. That this calendar-driven self-image is an artifice of culture is not permitted to have bearing on how we perceive ourselves. We give in to this self-image without thinking, as though the jolting acceleration into a new pattern is an inevitability.

What would life be like if we somehow had no way to mark the passage of years? How old would any of us think we were if we had no idea how old we were? We could not act our age if we did not know our age. We could not categorize ourselves into packaged groups of packaged interests and packaged capabilities. We would be much more what we really are: individuals of infinite variation at any age. The lockstep would end.

I am not arguing here for ignoring the passage of time. Nor am I suggesting an insensitivity to internal and surrounding reality. I am merely stating simple biological truth: We live in the biochemistry of our bodies, and not in years; we live in the interaction between that biochemistry and its greatest product—the human mind—and not in a series of decades marked by periodic lurches of change. Each of us exists therefore in a physical, mental, spiritual, and social individuality molded by everything that has come before and that is now brought to this moment of our lives. Each of us is the product of a cavalcade of living, whose sum is in every encounter in which we partake. Each of us is his or her own cohort. No number can define us as middle-aged, or elderly, or the oldest old. We can be defined only by what we have become. Whatever else aging may represent to us, it is first and foremost a state of mind.

And yet all of this is accompanied by that caveat, which needs reiteration here: Age does sometimes forget its own limitations, and inappropriately tries to be youth. Moments of sudden stress are known to encourage such behavior. Refusing to be hemmed in by a number does not mean the number is entirely without significance. Danger can lie in such unguarded spontaneity. Again, think of me, and the incident in the subway.

Many are the reasons for which we try to keep our bodies and minds at their optimal levels of functioning. Among the themes of the forthcoming chapters is the message that the ancient admonition of the Roman satirist Juvenal applies to all of us, no less at eighty than at eight, which becomes more meaningful with each passing year beyond forty. *Mens sana in corpore sano,* Juvenal advised, or as John Locke would put it a millennium and a half later in a treatise on the education of the young, "A sound mind in a sound body." But a foolish misapprehension of what is possible must not be allowed to lead one into error.

The danger of forgetting what should be expected of oneself is magnified when reserves have not been maintained, reserves that can respond to the unanticipated demands of everyday life. Though the full vigor of an earlier time is long gone, inner resources may burst forth when an older person has maintained a degree of fitness and self-confidence. We do not necessarily have to conform to society's traditional notion of what a man or woman should become when the middle years have been overtaken by the years associated in the minds of many with the downward arc of life's trajectory. I have several times been grateful that I have not been among the conformists, though a few episodes, like the one just described, have occurred because I have overreached, and forgotten to look down.

And so I am offering here what may seem to be a confusing mix of caution and advice: caution about the error of not looking down, and advice about one of the most crucial reasons for maintaining the physical and mental fitness that remains possible as we become older, namely, the possibility of having to call on powers whose use is rarely if ever necessary—whether in a situation of acute danger or in the case of illness. I do not mean to introduce or reveal ambivalence about the relative importance of looking up and looking down—both are equally important. Instead, what I do mean to introduce is the necessity to recognize that as we age, like at any other time of life, we must learn to live with contradictions—and not only contradictions, but uncertainties. The roadway is hardly clear as we attempt to find our way between retaining vigor and a realistic accommodation to its loss, any more than it has ever been clear in any previous era of our lives. That roadway is paved with uncertainty, and in this, too, each of us must find his or her own way, as we always have.

We elders maneuver through uncertainty by paying attention to our minds and bodies more carefully than ever in the past; we must make ourselves keen observers of their needs and their abilities. And in this, the developmental phase that we call aging is indeed different from those that preceded it. We are no longer at a stage where things will care for themselves; nothing can now be taken for granted. We have arrived at a time and place in our lives where we must study

ourselves as we have never done before, take care of ourselves, and be attuned to ourselves in ways that are new to us
and sometimes burdensome. This requires attention, reflection, and action, not only in regard to ourselves but in regard
to the world around us as well. In these ways, we older men
and women must all become philosophers.

TWO

HOW WE AGE:
BODY AND MIND

So accustomed have we become to the portrait of infirmity associated with nursing homes that many of us imagine it to be the norm, and a grim likeness of the waiting future: exhaustion to the point of listlessness, asthenia to the point of sickness, senility to the point of dementia. Visiting those grim holding pens for death, we have become familiar with their sights, sounds, and smells of incontinence, both physical and mental. These are the invariable colors in which life's final slow decline are commonly painted.

At the same time, each of us prefers to believe that he or she will somehow escape the catalogue of decrepitudes. No matter how close to our lives have been the acquaintances or relatives—including, sometimes, our own parents—who have succumbed to these decrepitudes' seeming inevitabilities, we cherish the conviction that we can avoid them, not only on account of some magical personal immunity, but also because times are changing so rapidly that such scenes of decline are fast fading from view. We tell ourselves that modern-day medical therapies and increasing knowledge of prevention are markedly lessening the likelihood that we will end our days in a way that Shakespeare's Jaques in *As You Like It* described as:

> . . . *second childishness and mere oblivion,*
> *Sans teeth, sans eyes, sans taste, sans everything.*

But despite reassurances, the specter of dotage does have a way of returning now and then to haunt our darker hours. Even the optimists seem at least occasionally beset by imaginings of themselves tottering unsteadily and oh so slowly toward the grave, finding their grim way by a flickering light barely recognizable as life. Alzheimer's, Parkinson's disease, strokes, cardiac crippling, and a generality of similar dwindlings—such are the fears that arise in the minds of those who allow themselves to ruminate on the possibility of end-stage affliction. We encounter the victims of these scourges everywhere, and it is sometimes impossible not to allow the intrusion of their images into one's own feared future.

Some of us are more resistant than others to such thoughts, but certain among us are virtually obsessed by them. In attempting to relax the hold these thoughts can have, it helps to know that relatively few of us will ever be confined to a nursing home. In the United States, only 4.5 percent of people over the age of sixty-five are denizened in such places, according to the 2000 census, and the number is gradually declining—in 1982, the figure was 6.3 percent. Not only is the number declining, but the average age of nursing home residents is going up, which means, at least in part, that people are entering such facilities later in life. The decrease in institutionalization may be used as an index of helpless debility in the general population; though plenty of old people are just as infirm in their own homes or the homes of their children, the general statistical trend of dependency appears to be downward, and there are good reasons for the decline.

Whatever other factors may have combined to decrease the frequency of infirmity and institutionalization (such as increased availability of assisted living facilities and adult day care), there seems little question that a changed attitude toward what had always been seen as inevitability has played a significant role. More of physiological loss than was previously realized falls into the category that might be called the atrophy of disuse, a concept clearly stated by Oliver Wendell Holmes more than 150 years ago: "Men do not quit playing because they grow old; they grow old because they quit playing." Recent clinical studies have confirmed Holmes's insight. We know important things nowadays about the role played by continued exercise of the body and mind in keeping our machineries running smoothly, whether they be joints, muscles, organs, or the cells and interconnections in our brains.

Advocates of one of several of the major schools of medical thought that existed in the seventeenth and eighteenth centuries called themselves iatromechanists (from the Greek *iatros*, physician) because they viewed the body as a vast machine made up of innumerable smaller machines. Their philosophy was expressed in a statement made by the Italian medical theorist Giorgio Baglivi in his 1704 book, *Opera omnia medico-practica et anatomica*:

Whoever examines the bodily organism with attention will certainly not fail to discern pincers in the jaws and teeth; a container in the stomach; water-mains in the veins, the arteries and other ducts; a piston in the heart; sieves or filters in the bowels; in the lungs, bellows; in the muscles, the force of the lever; in the corner of the eye, a pulley and so on. . . . It remains unquestionable that all these phenomena must be seen in the forces of the wedge, of equilibrium, of the lever, of the spring, and of all other principles of mechanics. In short, the natural functions of the living body can be explained in no other way so clearly and easily as by means of the experimental and mathematical principles with which nature herself speaks.

This simplistic view of bodily functioning would in later centuries be superseded by the realization of biochemical complexity and cellular dynamics, but it retains a certain metaphoric truth that has continued to appeal to scientists and teachers. The most popular small textbook on human structure and function during my medical student days in the 1950s bore the title *The Machinery of the Body*. Its authors, two physiologists named Anton Carlson and Victor Johnson, chose their title because it reflected with a certain clarity their sense of how best to convey an overall impression of the multitude of physical activities constantly at work within us. First published in 1930, the book required repeated printings of each of its five editions, culminating in the final one in 1961. Even today, a search on the Internet, under "The Machinery of the Body," lists what are described as "40 Million Books in One Web site. Used, New, Out of Print. Low Prices." The metaphor continues to be useful.

Especially in relation to running smoothly, the imagery of the body as machine will always apply. With respect to aging, the parallels are particularly apt: Aging parts work better when heed is paid to their maintenance; they require more attention than they did when they were new; they must be not only well cared for, but kept in active, albeit judicious, use.

Such analogies with machinery are hardly perfect, but they can nevertheless be carried just a bit further. As with machines, some human bodies are inherently built to last far longer than others, not only in respect to individual parts but pertaining also to their entire structure. In much the same way, inherited DNA influences longevity of each of our organs and the whole, but proper maintenance and appropriate use will maximize not only function but life expectancy as well.

The point is that individual men and women age at different rates, and much of the difference is dependent upon their inborn genetically determined constitution. Coming from a line of nonagenarians makes one prone to long life, for example, but does not guarantee it. There is, however, a flip side to this: Because of the way DNA does its somewhat haphazard mix-and-match, and because genes can express themselves in different ways depending on various internal and external influences, the predisposition to a long life not infrequently appears within a family whose members have been known to die early or at normative ages. Unfortunately, the opposite is true as well.

And also as with machines, a distinction must be made between parts that are frankly broken and parts that are merely showing the physical evidence of normal long usage. In regard to ourselves, it is important to recognize the distinction between aging and actual sickness. In some respects, this is no simple matter, even for physicians. But in other respects, the difference, once pointed out, is easily appreciated. Though aging does bring with it an increased vulnerability to certain illnesses, they are hardly its inescapable accompaniments. Aging is not a disease. It is a risk factor for many diseases—in the sense that older men and women are progressively less able to marshal the forces to withstand the encroachments of sickness—but it is not in itself a form of pathology.

Another way to look at the relationship between aging and disease is to imagine the later decades as a long continuum whose final destination is one or several named sicknesses—such as stroke, diabetes, or heart disease—but whose intervening points consist of relatively normal, though somewhat modified, functioning.

Stroke, for example, is a pathological condition, and not a normal consequence of aging. Its occurrence is made more likely by certain changes that are part of the ordinary growing older of blood vessels, but it is, most emphatically, a disease. Not only do the vast majority of people in their eighties and nineties not fall victim to strokes, but measures can often be taken to prevent strokes or lessen their effects, by applying awareness that their incidence increases with the passage of time. Alzheimer's, Parkinson's disease, coronary heart disease, cancer, diverticulitis, osteoporotic fractures—all of these and many more are examples of pathological conditions to which the older body is more prone than the younger, but which are nevertheless not to be expected as a consequence of normal aging.

Many men and women reach great age without sickness; more remarkably, many men and women reach great age without significant disability, though their machinery has lost some of its previous efficiency. For such men and women, the disease that finally comes along and kills them is likely to be of relatively short duration.

Everyone who has ever owned an automobile knows the importance of maintenance, but its application to the human body has become fully appreciated only within perhaps the last generation. In this as in all other considerations involving ourselves, biology is not necessarily destiny. Take, for example, the predisposition to obesity. Recent research indicates that obesity is largely determined by DNA. But despite that, it is also well known that lifestyle changes can modify—often substantially—what would appear to be the ordained consequence of heredity.

Sometimes, of course, the most scrupulous of maintenance will not add an hour to the life of an automobile whose parts are not built for long wear, but the opposite is far more likely to be the case: Taking good care of parts extends their usefulness and the usefulness of the whole machine. We now know this to be applicable to ourselves. Of the many reasons why a sixty-year-old of today looks, feels, and acts younger than a sixty-year-old of half a century ago, one is improved attention to upkeep.

Of all the factors that constitute human maintenance, improved methods of medical therapy appear to be among those of lesser importance, at least for any one individual. Responding to breakdown or its imminence is far less effective than prevention and attention to self-improvement, which have become increasingly recognized as the keys to healthy longevity. Even as the relentless inroads of time on our cells, tissues, and organs are taking place, their effects can be miti-

gated, slowed, and sometimes even reversed by proper attention to the kinds of maintenance that bodies routinely carry
out on their own when they are younger. There comes a stage
of life when we can no longer depend on the efficiency of nature's tendency to repair cellular irregularities and preserve
physiological balance. As this dependability lessens incre-
mentally throughout the middle years and later, we need
gradually to take over the job ourselves.

In the eighteenth and nineteenth centuries, a common
form of self-help manual was the so-called home medical
companion. In many households, such a volume was kept on
the shelf alongside a book consulted only slightly less frequently, the family Bible. Perhaps the best known and certainly the longest-lasting of these home therapy tomes was
William Buchan's *Domestic Medicine,* published in Edin-
burgh in 1769 and reprinted in scores of English and American versions. But my favorite of the genre, largely because of
its title and the fact that it was the first of its kind produced
in the United States, is a monograph written in 1734 by a
Tidewater physician named John Tennant, entitled *Every Man
his own Doctor.* This little handbook's subtitle described the
text's purpose: *Prescribing Plain and Easy Means for Persons
to cure themselves of all, or most of the Distempers, incident
to this Climate, and with very little Charge, the Medicines
being chiefly of the Growth and Production of this Country.*
If we are to assume the job of the body's maintenance ourselves, we can do no better than to use Tennant's title as an in-
spiration, for surely every man and woman can be his or her
own doctor, in the sense of being the maintenance person
who takes over the responsibility at which nature becomes
less adept as the sixth and seventh decades approach. Cer-

tainly, the kinds of habits and behaviors that will make such a difference in the quantity and quality of our lives conform in large portion to the criterion of being "Easy Means for Persons to cure themselves of all, or most of the Distempers, incident to this Climate, and with very little Charge."

In thinking about the ways in which personal behavior may influence the rate and degree of aging, it is useful to have some idea of the machinery itself, and the extent to which the passage of years is likely to affect individual parts of it. Though it has been emphasized that normal aging is not a disease, aging must nevertheless be seen as that long continuum whose eventual culmination is the disease that leads to death. The goal of an optimal lifestyle is to so slow down the process of this gradual change—the journey along the continuum—that reaching the threshold into sickness is long delayed.

Like all other generalized words, "aging"—whether in animals or man—is difficult to define with specificity. Nevertheless, all gerontologists—the scientists who study it—would agree that it is most usefully described as the process by which a healthy individual of any species gradually deteriorates into one that is frail, one whose bodily capacities and reserves are constantly diminishing at an ever-increasing rate, and one who is therefore becoming more and more vulnerable to disease and ultimate death. Though the tone of such a generic description sounds gravely pessimistic, what is actually experienced in the aging of human beings need hardly be so grim. The fact is that so little is yet known about the totality of factors that affect aging in any specific man or woman— not only with respect to organs, tissues, and the entire body, but even on the cellular and molecular level—that it is not at all clear that the progression is as relentless as such a generalized description makes it sound. Quite the contrary: Observations of large cohorts of older men and women provide strong evidence that the course of aging in humans is susceptible to modifying influences, some of which are within the control of each of us.

One of the reasons for the unpredictability in any individual human being is that so little is known about the interrelationships between the inherited genetic contributions to aging and those contributions that are either environmental or the result of what might be called an attitudinal response to the passing years. By this latter is meant that society has traditionally harbored lower physical and mental expectations for people older than sixty. In such an atmosphere of presumed decreased prospects, inactivity and sedentary habits become the norm, leading to a downward spiral of disuse and neglect of the very organ systems whose vibrancy is so necessary if debility and sickness are to be staved off. The consequence is deterioration into such problems as obesity, osteoporosis, hypertension, and chronic symptoms requiring drug therapy. Paradoxically, the very pharmaceuticals meant to mitigate debilitation may have side effects that in themselves lead to further decline. The interdependence of these four factors—normative genetic aging changes, disease, environmental influences, and decreased expectations resulting in inactivity of body and mind—are so complex that it is difficult to know what degree of influence each has as an independent variable. In any given man or woman, one or two of the factors may far outweigh the others. From numerous studies, it has become well known that higher activity levels correlate well with longer life spans. So much for the immutability of aging.

Even the seemingly inevitable normative—and genetically

determined—aging deteriorations appear less inevitable when they are closely examined. Such changes are in certain ways susceptible to modification, in response to modifications in our daily lives, and here is how:

The accumulation of errors in the regulation of gene function does lie at the basis of that portion of the aging process that is strictly biological. Some of these errors probably occur because they are predetermined by inherited controlling mechanisms—what might be called a "genetic tape"—that begins to run at conception and ends at death. Others are due to wear-and-tear factors in the environment within and around the cell as well as the environment within and around the entire body—such as diet, ultraviolet radiation, air pollutants, absorbed toxins like nicotine, and, very likely, stress. And, of course, time itself takes a toll. There is the decreasingly efficient removal from within the cell of toxic by-products of the cell's own metabolism; the cumulative oxidizing damage caused by the infamous free radicals; the occurrence of so-called cross-links between protein molecules that make them less flexible; the progressive collection of the yellow-brown pigment called lipofuscin within cells; the gradual aggregation of clumplike protein material, such as amyloid, in the extracellular fluid—and there are others. Such wear and tear affects not only genes, but protein molecules, biochemical interactions, and general cellular and organic function. To varying extents, we have some control over them.

Within each of our approximately seventy-five trillion cells, mechanisms exist to correct these errors as they occur, whether the errors are caused by relentless rolling of the genetic tape or by wear and tear. The longevity of any of us is largely determined by the ability of such cellular corrective mechanisms to counteract the baleful influence of time on our genetic functioning. But these mechanisms decline with age. As noted earlier, some of us are hereditarily better gifted for longevity than others, but all of us could be capable of helping our hereditary predisposition if only we knew how. Some of the "hows" that lie within the ability of all of us are well known. They consist of those lifestyles and environmental factors that maximize the cell's genetic battle against progressive deterioration. This means that we do have some control even at the level of our deepest biology.

One of the striking findings of research into the aging of the various organ systems of our bodies is the extreme variability between individuals. The brain, the liver, or the immune system, for example, of two people of the same age are often vastly different, with one person seeming much older than the other—much further along the continuum toward disease and death. Much of the difference is due to an inherited ability to recover from the various accumulated injuries to genetic integrity, but some of it is caused by the way an individual has lived his or her life, the environment in which one's life has been lived, and the attention paid to a healthy lifestyle—the amount of wear and tear, in other words. It is at the cellular and genetic level that we begin to find the way toward increased healthy longevity—but the cellular and genetic are influenced by the factors we encounter every day: diet, exercise, exposure to noxious agents, medications, and the like.

One example of the great individual variability of response to aging is found in the immune system, the body's complex of mechanisms that not only ward off infection but also play a large role in responding to the various agents that may cause cancer and autoimmune processes like rheumatoid arthritis and certain bowel diseases. Though the majority of the elderly have immunity that is 30 to 50 percent less than that of the young or middle-aged, some older people are able to mount an immune response almost as effectively as those much younger. Much of this responsiveness or lack of it is related to a person's general state of health, including such factors as nutrition, smoking, alcohol consumption, and environmental pollutants. The presence of intercurrent disease—what physicians call comorbidity—is also a factor, as are drugs and other medications used to treat it. So important are such influences that the ability to respond to assaults on the immune system is a good indicator of one's general state of health. The better shape we are in, the less prone we are to the condition that gerontologists call "immunosenescence"—senility of the immune system. The root *sen* is derived from the Latin *senex*, meaning "old man." No one wants to let his or her immune system become an old man.

Of all the parts of our bodies, the one in which the "let" of the previous sentence is most operative is surely the brain. The new research in neuroscience is demonstrating the remarkable ability of the human brain to influence its own aging. As astonishing as such a statement might at first seem, there is ever-increasing evidence of its validity, based not only on studies of cognition and behavior, but on equally revealing investigations into the structure and functioning of nerve cells, synapses, and the myriad networks of communications between far-flung parts of the central nervous system. Not only that, but the concept of mind—long a notion left for the most part to the ruminations of philosophers—is emerging as the object of scrutiny in the laboratories of our most talented scientists. It is no longer enough to conceive of mind as a function only of the brain; it must be thought of as influenced by the very factors that it has long been recognized to influence, namely, the body and our perceptions of the environment in which we find ourselves. In other words, the reciprocity of communication among the brain, the body, and what has been called "the econiche" in which we are situated determines the vast range of impressions and responses that go into the entirety of mind. As we mature, our exchange with the econiche becomes gradually more sophisticated, and the tree of knowledge and experience arborizes into a vast superstructure containing increasing numbers of reference points upon which incoming new material can adhere; the older brain is a huge and wide-ranging repository of information to which additional information is widely admitted because there are so many more points of entry as time passes and learning continues. In these ways, mind is often able to compensate for any organic capacity to perceive, learn, integrate, and use information that may be lost with advancing years. Brain may age, but mind continues to grow. Used well, an aging brain can become a more useful brain, and often a wiser one.

There can be no doubt that some organic capacity is indeed lost because of aging, but—assuming the absence of neurological or other comorbidity—such losses appear to be less than has long been presumed. There is unquestionably an approximate 5 percent decrease in brain weight and volume every ten years beyond the age of about forty, but some areas are relatively invulnerable to tissue loss. Because so much of the weight and volume loss consists of supporting tissue and the insulation around nerve fibers, rather than the cells' bodies, the meaning of the 5 percent figure is obscure. What is of realistic importance is not loss of substance in the sense of tissue but loss of substance in the sense of functioning. For this reason, the following discussion focuses on how the aging brain works rather than on which of its parts change in volume.

The fact is that modern methods of counting nerve cells (also called neurons) show no definite evidence of any but perhaps minimal age-related loss, except in the hippocampus—an area involved in emotional expression, learning, and memory—and selected locations in the cortex (the prefrontal and temporal-association areas), and only in certain parts of even these. In other words, the total number of brain cells in healthy older people decreases only slightly. But quality may influence these cells' effectiveness as much as quantity does. Like all other cells, those of the aging brain have been undergoing damage to proteins and metabolic processes throughout a long lifetime, as well as some slowing of cerebral blood flow. Decreased blood flow results in decreased metabolism of the oxygen and glucose so important in providing for the brain's enormous energy needs. It is likely that any losses in cognitive function are due to deficiencies in chemical neurotransmission rather than to any decrease in the number of neurons.

The cumulative result of such processes is lessened function, but the amount of lessening is so variable among individuals that it ranges from inconsequential to clinically troublesome. Among the several reasons why it may be inconsequential is redundancy, by which is meant that there is so much extra brain tissue that loss of some of it is without effect on function or intellectual capacity, since there are plenty of other nerves and fibers left to do the job. In addition, the same message may be transmissible over several distinct neural pathways, so that the loss of one of them merely means that a different course will be used thereafter.

Synapses are the connections between the fibers (called axons and dendrites) that extend from the bodies of nerve cells. Messages are carried across synapses—and therefore from one neuron to another—by means of chemicals called neurotransmitters. The cortex, the brain's convoluted outer mantle that does our thinking, contains some thirty billion nerve cells, and one million billion synapses by which these nerve cells interconnect with one another in myriad ways. The aging brain may have decreased numbers of synapses in some areas, but this is compensated by such factors as plasticity: the ability of synapses to become stronger and therefore more effective, to proliferate when required by neural activity, to enlarge in size, and to change configuration in response to altered patterns of usage. Loss of synapses in some areas is accompanied by no such loss in others, and is accompanied in some places by an increased number. In this as in so many other ways, the brain is always changing.

This ability to change is also demonstrable in the case of neurotransmitters and the receptors on the surface of nerve cells onto which they attach. While some neurotransmitters and some receptors decrease with age, others increase, with the result that certain cerebral functions may be lessened, certain may be heightened, and certain may remain unaffected. Also, cell loss is at least in part compensated by the production of new cells, as has been discovered only in the past decade. Prior to this discovery, it was believed that no such process was possible in the central nervous system.

The result of the competing and balancing influences of gain and loss manifests itself in how effectively the brain functions in any given individual. The following paragraphs should be considered a general summation of what occurs in normative healthy aging, realizing that variability is so great that far more than a few older men and women continue into extreme old age with minimal or even no demonstrable loss of cerebral ability.

It is true that learning is somewhat slower, and the amount learned with the same effort and exposure lessens, as the later years progress. But the ability to assimilate information and to learn from experience does not change appreciably. Perhaps as important to acquiring new knowledge, attention does not become impaired. Though verbal abilities do not decrease, creative thinking and problem-solving abilities slowly decline. This means that intellectual quickness and on-the-spot reasoning slow; mental agility is the province of the young. As Sir Francis Bacon put it three centuries before brain scanning had become so much as a possibility on the horizon, "Young men are fitter to invent than to judge, fitter for execution than for counsel, and fitter for new projects than for settled business."

Not only is intellectual quickness impaired with aging but so is reaction time. Aging increases reaction time because the process of cognition—the awareness and instantaneous processing of information—is somewhat slowed, as is the peripheral motor response to stimuli. Ordinarily, these changes are perceptible only under conditions of immediacy, but modern living means that immediacy is everywhere, and especially behind the wheel of an automobile going seventy miles an hour in a rainstorm at night. As drivers get into their seventies and beyond, they should choose their traveling times and conditions with increasing circumspection.

The cognitive complaint most often made by or about older men and women is loss of memory. Though long-term memory (and sensory memory too, of smells, tastes, and sounds) is not significantly disrupted—nor is vocabulary and the general store of culture- and education-based information—short-term memory is more likely to become a problem, even under the physiological conditions of healthy aging. And yet, some nonagenarians continue with memory so unimpaired as to be comparable to that of a young adult. Such a circumstance is usually the reflection of a general state of cerebral function that has remained at a high level for all parameters of activity.

At the beginning of this discussion, reference was made to the brain's ability to influence its own aging. The evidence for this comes from several disparate sources. One source of evidence is the observation that the frequency of Alzheimer's disease and other dementias appears to be somewhat less in people who have pursued an active intellectual life. Another source of evidence is the discovery in the laboratory of a class of protein substances that have the ability to protect neurons against injury and death, as well as the ability to stimulate the production of new neurons from adult stem cells in the brain. It has been demonstrated in cell culture and in rodents that the production and effectiveness of these protein substances, called neurotrophic (nerve growth) factors, is determined by the amount of activity going on in nearby neural circuits; the more the circuits are used, the more neurotrophic factor is produced. This means not only that lost, damaged, or impaired nerve cells can be replaced, but also that an increased population of new nerve cells may occur in certain locations in the brain. It is now clear that there is a demonstrable biochemical reason—the increase in various neurotrophic factors, which are a result of increased cerebral activity—why using our brains is likely to increase the number and effectiveness of neurons. This evidence substantiates the everyday observation that those who continue to challenge themselves intellectually are likely to be those who maintain the capacity to do so.

The production of one of these protein substances, brain-derived neurotrophic factor, or BDNF, is increased not only by cerebral activity but also by aerobic exercise, and a few more words will be said about this later in the book. For now, it is enough to point out that the joggers you are accustomed to seeing or accompanying through the streets and byways of your community are doing far more than merely burning calories and improving their cardiovascular function. They are improving their minds as well, just as if they were reading a volume of Aristotle. Joggers, readers, thinkers, and doers of every stripe are influencing the aging process and healthy functioning of the human brain by taking advantage of its ability to change with use, and ever to expand its possibilities.

But of course, the joggers are doing their thing because they want to increase the capacity of their cardiovascular systems, probably not realizing how much smarter they are getting while huffing and puffing in the interests of staving off the aging changes that are trying to overtake their hearts and blood vessels. Those changes are far less complex than the ones trying to make headway in the brain. Though the frequencies of arteriosclerosis and hypertension are generally high in the elderly, many people reach their eighties and nineties with little or no disease of the heart or major arteries. As with all other parts of the body, there is great variation in how an individual's heart and arteries may be affected by aging, ranging from the barely affected to the severely compromised. The following description pertains to what the average person can expect.

Perhaps more than is true for most systems other than the brain, lifetime habits are crucial determinants of the condition of one's heart and arteries. Not unexpectedly, the most profound influences are due to those well-known factors—here they come again—of diet, obesity, smoking, physical activity, cholesterol level, and personality. Chronic diseases, of which hypertension and diabetes are among the most prominent, also play a major and often determining role.

In the absence of significant comorbidity, the aging heart and blood vessels manage astonishingly well. They are able to compensate so effectively for the normal anatomic and physiologic alterations of the years that, under ordinary circumstances, there is neither decrease in cardiac output nor abnormality of heart rate when at rest or when engaging in non-stressing activities. Among those normal alterations of aging are a gradual loss of elasticity in the major vessels, particularly the aorta, which is the large artery leading directly out of the heart. This decreased elasticity—caused in large part by the aggregation of protein strands into the cross-links mentioned earlier—causes the aorta to become wider and to elongate somewhat, thereby adding to its dimensions and forcing the heart to work harder in order to drive blood through its greater capaciousness. At first, the heart can compensate quite well for the increased work without raising the blood pressure required to do the job, but this begins to change slowly at about age sixty. Around this time, the heart begins to enlarge a bit, and the average systolic (upper number) blood pressure starts creeping upward from a normal of approximately 120 to a level of 140 for a healthy seventy-year-old.

Such numbers can merge into the pathological range, so that 15 percent of Caucasians and 25 percent of African Americans are hypertensive by the time they are sixty-five. Beyond that age, the figure is 1 in 4 for Caucasians and 1 in 3 for African Americans. Some surveys provide figures even higher than these. Of the several reasons why the increased pressure is dangerous, one is its tendency to cause damage to the lining of small blood vessels in the brain, leading to such problems as cognitive defects, stroke, and dementia.

In a normally aging heart, increasing amounts of fibrous tissue gradually begin to appear between the organ's muscle cells, which are themselves slowly decreasing in number, so that by age seventy about a third of these muscle cells have been lost. At the same time, the number of the heart's nerve cells, and their interconnecting fibers, is going down, so transmission of the electrical signals that trigger the heartbeat becomes less efficient, causing the organ to slow somewhat with age and eject less blood with each passing year.

Despite these losses, the mechanisms continue to function well so long as they are not subjected to stress. The older organ's difference from a younger, normal heart is not apparent unless a challenge of some sort takes place, such as the need to run in order to catch a train, or perhaps the sudden emotional upheaval of anxiety or anger. In such situations, the aging ventricles are not able to accommodate efficiently.

For example, older people are not nearly as able to vary their heart rate as they were when they were younger. Accordingly, the heart rate cannot increase as rapidly or as much in response to exercise. Also, after the rate does become elevated, it takes longer to return to baseline level. (A good rule of thumb is that 220 minus one's age is the maximum heart rate that can be attained with vigorous exercise.) This means that the heart's output is adapting less effectively than it once did to sudden needs that may be imposed on it.

It is for these reasons that a continued high level of activity is so important. Cardiac efficiency under conditions of stress can be markedly improved by exercise training. A heart that has been benefited by a consistent schedule of vigorous exertion can respond to stress like a heart several decades younger, not only by its added ability to beat more forcefully and faster, but also by the capacity of its muscle cells to take up the required supplemental supply of oxygen from the blood. This ability is aided by the effect of an exercise program on the chest wall. Because the chest wall becomes stiffer with age and its muscles weaken, general respiratory function lessens. But these changes are to a significant extent reduced by a vigorous program of aerobic exercise, which provides the added oxygen required by the stressed heart.

Exercise training also contributes other benefits for the cardiovascular system. Training improves the ability of the larger arteries to adapt to the heightened blood flow required by exertion, and it increases the sensitivity of certain pressure-monitoring structures—called baroreceptors—in the arterial walls. This is particularly important because normal aging causes (1) a decrease in blood flow through the thickening and less elastic middle-size arteries such as those to the kidney and liver; (2) a lessening of the number of capillaries throughout the body; (3) a narrowing in the diameter of the larger veins; and (4) a thickening and loss of elasticity of the heart's valves, as well as some deposition of calcium in the valves' leaflets. And, of course, the extent of arteriosclerosis—hardening of the arteries—is imperceptibly increasing all the time. Improved biological self-monitoring of pressure and flow leads to improved responsiveness in these structures when stress occurs. Planned vigorous exercise is a far better anti-aging treatment than all the elixirs, creams, lotions, potions, and cosmetic surgery in the world.

The various cardiac and vascular alterations described in the foregoing paragraphs occur even in the absence of any significant arteriosclerosis or hypertension. The addition of either of these pathologies results in worsening cardiovascular function, depending on the degree to which the pathology is present. But even under such circumstances of disease, response to stress can be improved with carefully graded exercise programs. Clearly, the physical workouts of men or women who have suffered heart attacks require meticulous oversight by their physicians. This is true not only on account of the danger of overstress but also because the older coronary arteries have lost some of their ability to make new collateral vessels to replace those that have become obstructed. This formation of new vessels is called angiogenesis.

But the most remarkable characteristics of the cardiovascular system's response to aging are the two already mentioned, which it shares with all other organs and tissues of the body: its extreme variability from one person to another and its continuing competence to do its job perfectly well under normal conditions, even when it can no longer deal as effectively with major challenges.

Another example of this sort of thing is found in the functioning of the body's hormones and the structures that produce them, called endocrine glands. Here too certain of the aging changes occur to varying degrees in virtually everyone, while others of the aging changes are less universal. The first category involves a decreased ability of the intestine to absorb calcium, and so the amount of that mineral in the blood tends to become lower. In an attempt to keep the level steady, the parathyroids—glands buried deep within the thyroid, whose function is to control calcium metabolism—raise their output of hormone (called parathyroid hormone, or PTH), which has the effect of drawing calcium out of the bones and into the bloodstream. The lowered concentration of calcium in the bones worsens osteoporosis, which is already being caused by a combination of (1) certain aging changes in the cells that manufacture bone and (2) the loss of significant numbers of these cells. The decreased bone density that is the result of these two factors produces few or no symptoms unless the decrease becomes advanced. Because men have higher bone density than women and also because postmenopausal deficiency of estrogen causes bone loss (the reasons why are unclear), osteoporosis tends to be more severe in women, though men are hardly free of varying degrees of it, sometimes to the point of debility. Depending on the criteria for its diagnosis, about a third of men beyond the age of seventy-five are found to have osteoporosis. Not only the severity but the frequency of osteoporosis is more marked in women, by a factor that some estimate to be as high as 4 to 1. As with the body's other aging mechanisms, individual variation results in a wide spectrum of how a person may be affected by this condition.

One's position on that spectrum is influenced by physical activity. The more stress put on a bone by the forces of the muscle attached to it, the more its cells respond by doing all they can to maintain and even add to bone mass and strength, including increasing the absorption of calcium from the bloodstream. Just as a sedentary life encourages the loss of bone, a vigorously active life encourages increase in bone density.

Like disease of the cardiovascular system, loss of bone density can be managed by a variety of means in addition to exercise; the choice depends on the cause or causes thought to be most significant. Oral supplements of calcium and the vitamin D that increases calcium's absorption from the intestine should be a standard part of the daily diet, beginning perhaps in one's early fifties. The vitamin D becomes more important with the passing of years, to counteract the age-associated decrease of the vitamin in the body.

Because age-related loss of bone density is ultimately the result of a complex of changes at the level of the cell's ability to make new bone, it is particularly important to combat the loss in the ways just described, with the addition of estrogen replacement therapy for women so long as there are no contraindications to its use in any given individual. Of course, other therapies of a pharmaceutical nature are available should osteoporosis become severe enough to require treatment, including those that bind with estrogens and influence their activity.

Though all of the body's systems lose elements of function

as the years pass, it is in the muscles and bones that major problems are likely to be most frequent, and these problems are almost as obvious as such developments are in an organ as visible as the skin. Among the most obvious changes is the decrease in muscle and the increase in fat. Musculoskeletal inadequacy is the single most common cause of debility in the old. Largely because of a decreased ability to manufacture the necessary protein, muscle mass lessens, a process that speeds up after the age of fifty. But contractile force decreases out of proportion to that change, probably as a result of some general alteration in neural signaling and coordination of fibers. By age sixty-five or seventy, about one-third of muscle strength has been lost, with loss becoming more rapid as the years add up. This seems to be due to a combination of fewer muscle fibers, the decreased size of each fiber, and a lessened ability of the fibers to function in a coordinated manner. As will be discussed later in this book, strength can be improved markedly with weight training, so much so that the muscle strength of a determined older man or woman can often be brought to a level comparable to that of a much younger person.

Falls become an increasingly important source of disability as people get older. Falls happen not only because of decreased strength and coordination but also because of a lessened range of joint motion and because of a generally decreased reaction time. All of these factors are accentuated by the kinds of neurologic deficits that sometimes make walking so hazardous. Improvements in coordination, muscle strength, and reaction time not only make falls less common, but also have the added benefit of increasing the likelihood that one will be able to control a fall sufficiently to lower the probability of fracturing a bone or dislocating a joint.

Here it seems appropriate to insert a parenthetical word about alcohol intake. Though strong evidence exists that the consumption of small to moderate amounts of alcohol, especially red wine, exerts protective effects on the incidence of strokes, coronary heart disease, gallstones, infections, and even the common cold, this should not be interpreted as a warrant to drink beyond such reasonable amounts. In the elderly, even the smallest degree of tipsiness markedly increases the frequency of falls and fractures, which means that a degree of circumspection and prudence is required each time a drink is considered. Not only that, but just a bit of euphoria impairs the judgment required to safely drive a car, especially for the elderly. These caveats are complicated by the fact that older drivers are more likely to be seriously injured than their younger counterparts experiencing similar types of auto accidents. And, of course, they are less likely to recover. In addition, one should account for the possibility of harmful interactions with the drugs that people beyond certain ages are more likely to be taking. The time for judgment is *before* drinking and not when it is too late.

Just as the preservation or rebuilding of muscle and bone are to a considerable extent determined by relatively simple measures, their opposites—loss of density and strength—are to a considerable extent determined by expectations. If one's image of aging involves an inactive and generally sedentary existence, his or her punishment will be unnecessary loss of muscle and bone, leading to even less activity; if one's image of aging involves vigorous participation in a variety of enthusiasms, his or her reward will be a gain of muscle and bone, allowing even more activity. In such ways, assumptions about the aging process become self-fulfilling prophecies.

The decreased estrogen levels that contribute to osteo-porosis and other problems in postmenopausal women ap-pear relatively rapidly. Men, on the other hand, lose testicular function gradually—so gradually that some men never be-come markedly deficient. Occasional octogenarians and even nonagenarians continue to have blood levels of testosterone that would be normal for a young adult. Unfortunately, this does not necessarily translate into retained libido and sexual potency.

Libido and sexual potency—has there ever been a man who did not give a thought to their decline with the years? Has there ever been a woman who did not wonder whether her libido or lack of it was "normal" for her age? Cicero, in his oft-quoted dissertation on aging, *de Senectute,* disposed of the entire matter by asserting that older people are well rid of their need for sensual pleasure, which "is a foe to reason, and, so to speak, blinds the eyes of the mind." At the age of sixty-three, he felt himself happy to be free of its demands. "Far from being a charge against old age, that it does not much feel the want of any [sexual] pleasures, it is its highest praise." Today, far fewer would agree with the Roman sage than protest that he had things all wrong. Though many el-derly men and women feel that their sexuality is a thing of the past, many more continue to be active or continue to wish hopefully that circumstances allowed them to partake of what Cicero called a "deadly curse."

Statistics about sexual behavior in the older population are hard to come by (no pun is here intended, and certainly not a double one) and notoriously unreliable. There are nu-merous reasons for this, but suffice it to say that no one should become discouraged by statements either of continued desire and activity or of the opposite: lack of interest or ability to achieve any degree of satisfaction. Not only is there vast unreliability in the design of published studies done by surveys and suppositions, but even those experts most skilled in various areas of geriatric science and sociology seem to lose themselves in enthusiastic encouragement when writing about sex. An example of this is found in the standard academic text in the specialty of geriatrics and its associated research, a perfectly wonderful 1648-page volume compiled by five distinguished editors and no fewer than 207 authoritative contributors. Few would disagree that there is no more useful or reliable volume on the clinical and scientific aspects of the subject than *Principles of Geriatric Medicine & Gerontology*. But the second sentence of the book's chapter entitled "Sexuality and Aging" unequivocally states, "It is reassuring to know that aging itself does not lead to sexual problems." The chapter's two authors—one of whom is, with very good reason, among the world's most highly respected leaders in the field of aging—then go on to describe (with the clarity and wisdom that characterizes all of their other writings) all manner of obstacles to the kind of sexual functioning to which most men and women are accustomed during their earlier years.

It seems apparent from reading any significant amount of the pertinent medical literature and from virtually everyone's personal experience that sex at seventy is a very different thing from sex at thirty-five, or even at sixty. And there are plenty of physiological reasons for the differences. The most obvious ones are related to the general lessening of male hormone levels in men and the marked decline of female hormones in women. Though an occasional elderly man, as noted above, is found to have testosterone levels equivalent to those of a thirty-year-old, such a thing is highly unusual and its significance uncertain. As for estrogens, they drop steeply during menopause. These and other physiological manifestations of aging have significant consequences for both desire and the nature of activity. To not call them problems is to deny their very real effect on lovemaking.

For women, some degree of thinning of the vaginal wall is inevitable, as is variable loss of the vagina's length, width, and elasticity, as well as lessened lubrication, especially during sexual activity. Such changes may make intercourse difficult, uncomfortable, and sometimes painful, even when a bit of bleeding is not caused by local injury during thrusting. The labia lose firmness as they age, the fatty mound over the pubis (classically called the mons veneris, the mound of love) flattens, and the pubic hair becomes sparser. The entire appearance of the field of lovemaking for females has thus become altered.

For men, an erection is slower to begin and to reach its peak. From the instant or two previously required to make itself evident, the time extends to increasing numbers of minutes, and in a significant percentage approaches infinity, in the sense that all the waiting or manual stimulation in the world has no effect; impotence has reared its flaccid head. The erection of the aging penis often does not become as hard, as large, or as long-lasting as it once was. Orgasms, when they occur, are usually less explosive, take a longer time to come forth, and require far more time to repeat themselves, sometimes measurable in days or weeks. As for fertility, some men have fathered children in their nineties, but most have become sterile by the time they are seventy-five.

Authors seem to shy away from saying anything about the appearance of aging male genitals, but one need not have done thousands of physical exams in a long career of surgery—it is necessary only to spend the most minimum time in the locker rooms of athletic clubs—to verify that an older penis usually appears somewhat droopier and perhaps a bit smaller than the fuller, younger ones nearby. Its companion testicles hang lower than they did years ago, because of loss of turgor in the skin muscle of the scrotum, a muscle called the dartos. As in the female, the pubic hair is less dense and has lost some of its curl. Altogether, the elderly male sexual apparatus does not present the image of bursting virility that was once its hallmark.

Desire and what some sex manuals unfortunately call "performance" for both men and women result from a complex of physiological, sensory, and emotional factors that must act in delicately balanced concert if satisfaction is to be achieved. It stands to reason that the neurological, vascular, hormonal, and other physical aspects of this mix will be less efficient with age, as is the coordination required to make everything function with the perfection of timing so necessary to the desired result. In such a situation, inhibiting psychological factors take on a significance at least as great as they did in youth, when a certain animal automaticity of response may have helped to overcome them.

Older women worry about being unattractive because of wrinkles or sagging flesh, and they may be concerned about the possibility of sexual discomfort or unresponsiveness. Older men are more likely to distress themselves with fears of insufficient libido or of impotence. Both partners bring an entire lifetime of attitudes toward and experience with sexuality that influences their approach to lovemaking. When they are married or in some other form of long-term relationship, these matters may be eased, but hardly always. Men and women, whether straight or gay, are not infrequently inhibited in new sexual relationships by an assortment of factors that stand in the way of fulfillment. In general, the patterns of late-life sexuality reflect the patterns of the decades that preceded them.

There is no way to know what is sexually "normal" at any time of life, and the older years are more resistant to the word's definition than any others. Even more than is true of the effects of aging on all other functions and structures of the body, the variability in sexual activity, ability, and satisfaction is enormous. Some few men and women are as active as they were at much younger ages, and many others are far less so but nevertheless quite satisfied with what is possible for them, though it may involve methods short of actual coitus, such as cuddling and mutual masturbation. Still others are without sexual activity at all, because of attitudes about aging, lack of appropriate partners, loss of desire, medical problems of various sorts, choice based on social constraints, or any of an assortment of other factors. The ultimate question about the sexuality of older men and women is whether they are content with what they have. And here perhaps the authors who deny the existence of problems deserve more consideration than I at first gave them. The problems, as always in the eye of the beholder, do exist for many of the elderly, but useful solutions are available for some of them. For the others and for the entire spectrum of sexual relationships among older men and women, we might turn to Shakespeare for the most appropriate response, when he has

Hamlet say, "There is nothing either good or bad, but think-ing makes it so."

When the participants feel discontented with their sexual life, it is almost always because it is not of the quality or quantity they might wish for. Especially because most of the very real problems associated with the sexuality of aging in-dividuals has been found to be physical—and not emotional, as was previously thought—such men and women should be encouraged to seek medical help, because so many of their difficulties are now being treated with increasing success.

Just as is the situation for sexuality and the physical ele-ments involved—as well as the heart, parathyroids, ovaries, and testicles—all other glands and organs lose elements of function as they become older, and they do so in a variety of ways. The thyroid, for example, tends to slow its function of regulating the rate of metabolism—but not very much. The incidence of levels of thyroid activity in the elderly so low as to be of consequence is less than 10 percent. The insulin-secreting cells of the pancreas, on the other hand, are more likely to cause trouble. The resultant diabetes often goes un-recognized and undiagnosed in elderly people, and therefore untreated.

The two major sensory organs, the eye and ear, likewise vary considerably among individuals as they age. Predictably, decreased flexibility in the lens of the eye results in loss of ability to accommodate and focus for near vision, explaining the frequency of bifocals on the noses of people beginning at about age forty-five. In addition, adaptation to dark becomes more difficult, which, when combined with an increased sen-sitivity to glare, makes many older men and women prefer to not drive at night. The problems with glare are the reason that elders are more often than younger people likely to be seen wearing tinted glasses indoors. Even relatively minor manifestations of decreased accommodation and ability in adapting to dark make the possibility of stumbling greater. Should there be any significant degree of the opacification of the lens so common in people on their way to a cataract, the tendency to lose one's footing or to fall is obviously more pronounced. Though cataract is the most common of the serious visual impairments to which they are prone, the elderly also have a higher incidence of glaucoma, macular degeneration, and diabetic pathology of the retina.

The tendency toward the development of cataracts is increased among smokers, diabetics, men and women with a history of long exposure to sunlight, and those who have required cortisone-like compounds for extensive periods, but other than the general process of protein fibers conglomerating into cross-links, not much is known about the biochemical basis for the development of cataracts. They are so common that surgery to correct them is the most frequent of the major operations covered by Medicare.

In reference to what is "the most common," it will surprise no one who has ever had to raise his voice while speaking with an elderly uncle that the most common of all chronic health issues among men over sixty-five is significant hearing loss; though somewhat less frequent among women, it is nevertheless a problem hardly restricted to the aging male. Lifelong exposure to noise worsens a difficulty that is due primarily to degeneration in the auditory nerve and in the cochlea, the snail-shaped inner ear structure that contains the essential organs of hearing. But here, too, variations among individuals can be enormous, especially since the decibel level in which people live and work varies so widely. Incidentally, another of the reasons not to smoke is the increased likelihood of hearing loss that occurs in the later years among those who do.

By now, there have appeared in this chapter enough warnings about the dangers of smoking that they may have become tedious. Nevertheless, be prepared for another one, which I can best illustrate by describing the most useful method I have ever discovered to influence my patients to quit cigarettes. Early in my surgical practice, I began to notice that there was a particular clue that was virtually foolproof in identifying a heavy smoker immediately on greeting her in the consulting room, and it was as plain as the nose on her face. I have chosen "her" rather than "him" to describe the phenomenon because this particular bit of evidence is more noticeable in women, and somewhat less obvious in men. I refer here to a specific pattern and distribution of very fine wrinkling that gradually merges into a greater degree of coarseness as the years of not kicking the habit go on and on. The hair-thin lines appear first in the skin at the corners of the mouth, and then advance with time to involve the area below the nostrils and laterally on the cheeks, as well as the corners of the eyes—the so-called crow's-feet. The more delicate the skin over any particular location, the more wrinkling occurs. Barely noticcable in their early years—which are usually the late thirties or early forties—these lines progress over perhaps a decade until it is impossible not to be aware of them once their significance is known. They look quite different from the usual subtle aging changes that begin to make their appearance at this age, and become even more obviously different as time passes. By the fifties, the skin of a moderate to heavy smoker's face has taken on features that are unmistakable, and looks more weather-beaten and older than her non-smoking sister's. Simply stated, the face of a middle-aged smoker looks older than the face of an abstainer.

Every experienced physician knows that fear of cancer, emphysema, or any of the other serious problems that a smoker's flesh is heir to convinces few relatively young people to give up cigarettes. And so it became my custom, immediately after the introductory smile and greeting, to ask suspect new patients a single brief question: "Why do you smoke so much?" When my suspicions proved correct, which was almost always, the response was in most cases an alarmed glance and some variant of "How can you tell?" Though I have no statistics, I do know that I started far more smokers—particularly women—on the road to abstinence by this appeal to vanity than I ever succeeded in doing by invoking the specter of disease.

Some years after initially making this observation, I began to find reports in medical literature confirming it, and suggesting reasons why the wrinkling occurs. Apparently, the tiny arteries supplying the skin of the face are particularly susceptible to the narrowing effects of nicotine, both acutely with the spasm caused by each cigarette and chronically with the gradual buildup of obstructing material on the arteries' lining, which effectively obliterates them. The cumulative result is loss of blood supply, most manifest in the finer parts of the skin. A smoker at sixty looks like an abstainer at seventy.

Though smoking does worsen almost all of them, other aging changes in the skin—which, by the way, is our largest organ—are less under our control. The one exception is the ultraviolet irradiation of the sun, about which most of us can do a great deal. Unlike chronological aging, which is directly proportional to time, so-called photoaging is more related to level of skin pigment and degree of exposure. And it is also unlike chronological aging in the appearance that results from it. The appearance of chronological aging tends to be skin that is pale, smooth, and finely wrinkled, whereas the appearance of photoaging is more commonly skin that is coarsely wrinkled, darker in color, and often disfigured by spidery superficial blood vessels and brownish blotches as well as occasional superficial thickenings, some of which are in fact premalignant lesions. Since the fundamental molecular changes for both conditions have been shown to share certain characteristics, it behooves all of us, and particularly those with light-colored skin, to avoid direct sunlight as much as possible, and at appropriate times to take advantage of the various highly effective sunscreens now available.

The skin is in a sense the show window of our years, and we tend to watch with dismay as it becomes wrinkled, lax, and less resilient with time. The wrinkling occurs because col-lagen, the protein fiber that maintains firmness, is gradually lost; the same is true of elastin, the protein responsible for flexibility and, as its name implies, elasticity. Other compounds with the forbidding name of glycosaminoglycans keep the skin moist and supple by binding with water. Because all of these materials dwindle with time, the skin becomes dryer, thinner, and less buoyant, as does its underlying layer of fatty tissue, whose function is to protect the skin by a cushioning effect. Skin loses its former ability to recoil, an effect abetted by the same process of cross-linking among adjacent protein strands that promotes cataract formation in the eye and loss of elasticity in arteries. The number of nerve endings, sweat glands, microscopic feeding blood vessels, and pigment cells decreases. Accordingly, the skin is more prone to injury and delayed healing, factors that make the skin of the very elderly prone to sores, ulceration, and infection. These effects are most pronounced in body areas where the surface is thinnest, such as the face, hands, ankles, and tops of the feet. The scanter fatty layer, lessened circulation, and smaller number of sweat glands compromise the skin's function of stabilizing body temperature, so the elderly are particularly prone to heatstroke, the effects of cold, and other manifestations of suboptimal surrounding conditions. Even healthy people beyond age sixty should be aware of such matters, and take account of them in tending to their general well-being—and their show window. But certain caveats are in order at any age beyond youth. Among them is that cigarettes and sunshine may cause cancer only in certain unlucky individuals, but we can be sure that their effects on all of us are universal: By prematurely aging the skin, they not only compromise our attempts to appear younger, but make us look older than we are.

Unlike in organs such as the skin, aging changes in the kidney are relatively independent of anything we can do to lessen or accelerate them. The kidneys are yet another example of structures that continue to perform quite well in the great majority of people so long as they are not subjected to inordinate challenge. Among other manifestations of their loss of reserve capacity is a lessened tolerance to the intake of excessive salt or water. In all, approximately 20 percent of the elderly have some significant degree of kidney impairment, but only in one-quarter to one-half of these (amounting to 5 to 10 percent of the entire elderly population) is it marked. In other individuals, the normative aging changes—decreased kidney weight, scarring of the filtering units, and a lowering of blood flow to an eventual level of about half of what it was in young adulthood—have little effect on ordinary functioning unless hypertension, diabetes, or some other chronic or acute disease is present. Such illnesses decrease kidney function, and so may the pharmaceutical agents used to treat them.

The aspect of the urinary tract that does tend to let some people—though far from the majority—down is the ability to control and pass urine. Because the aging bladder loses some distensibility, its capacity lessens and urination is more frequent. The situation is not helped by the onset of varying degrees of discoordination between the bladder muscle that pushes urine out and the finely tuned shutter mechanism that helps to keep it in, which must relax at precisely the right instant if all is to go well. A complicating factor may derive from the muscular and fibrous structures of the pelvic floor, which aid in the suspension of the bladder. These sometimes weaken with age, particularly in women who have had several children. This may lead to the annoyance called stress incontinence, perhaps best exemplified by the fortyish mother of three who, on being told a particularly funny story, is said to have laughed and laughed until she felt a little run-down. The muscular and fibrous weakening adds to the tendency toward major problems with incontinence that are experienced by certain of the elderly, particularly those who are somewhat debilitated. Incontinence and retention may contribute to infection, which in turn is an aggravating factor to both problems, as are mental confusion, certain medications, and an enlarged prostate.

Enlargement of the prostate is caused by aging changes in the complex relationship between the sex hormones and the cellular and fibrous components of the gland. Because the greatest resultant proliferation of cells occurs in the region around the urethra, some degree of hindrance of the urinary stream occurs in many men. The symptoms, which occur in approximately 30 percent of men, vary from occasional difficulty in beginning to void, all the way to complete obstruction, which requires some sort of medical intervention.

Unlike the kidneys, the aging gastrointestinal tract is likely to become the source of symptoms of various kinds, though here, too, there is great variability among individuals. Acid reflux, constipation, diverticulitis, gallstones, swallowing abnormalities, susceptibility to bacterial gastroenteritis, decreased sphincter reliability, hemorrhoids—all of these are far more likely to plague the old than the young. But some of these changes are not, strictly speaking, due to age. Instead, they are caused—or at least abetted—by the generally sedentary patterns into which older people too commonly lapse. Many allow themselves to become far less mobile than they once were, to ingest fewer liquids and dietary fiber, and to take more questionably necessary medications, which may worsen any propensities to gastrointestinal problems. Of course, older people's increased frequency of comorbid disease also worsens such propensities. The solution to some, but obviously not all, of these problems is often found in the greater activity that is the product of not thinking of oneself as over the hill.

Because much of the energy generated by exercise is a factor in raising body temperature, decreasing activity may be the reason why the body temperature of older people is likely to be lower than it was in middle age. Modern studies indicate that the nineteenth century benchmark of 98.6 degrees for a young adult should be lowered to the more accurate 98.2, but the body temperature is lower still as the elder decades are reached. The average midday temperature for eighty-year-olds living independently is probably in the neighborhood of 97.7, though it fluctuates as much as a degree during the course of a normal day, as it does for people in all age categories. The 97.7 figure means that the definition of what constitutes a fever must be reinterpreted by about half a degree when dealing with men and women beyond the age of seventy-five. The problem is further complicated by the fact that the fever response to inflammation and infection, like all of the body's other responses to stress, may lessen with age. Accordingly, it is not uncommon for the sick elderly to not exhibit a significant rise in body temperature even when quite ill.

Ultimately, scientists still know far less about the biology of aging than they would like to. In many respects, it remains a great mystery, just as life itself is a great mystery. But we live it with the knowledge we have, just as we must face aging with the knowledge we have. And despite all uncertainties, there are matters we already understand very well. One of them is the principle of maintenance, the principle that John Tennant called *Plain and Easy Means* in his self-help manual of 1734. Though there is much in our bodies and in our susceptibility to disease and aging that we will never be able to control, we yet have far more influence on aspects of these processes than has until recently been realized. Not to use that influence is to allow oneself to succumb to an unjustified resignation that has marred and shortened the lives of generations of our forebears; not to use that influence is to invite debility, disease, and death.

THREE

APPROACHING A CENTURY: MICHAEL DEBAKEY

In matters of longevity, a certain very few men and women not only have outdone the vast majority of humankind, but have made such good use of their extra years that they are a wonderment to the rest of us. These are people who stride through their ninth and tenth decades with much the same enthusiasm and productivity that characterized their fifth or sixth. We would all like to emulate them, but nature and reality dictate that only a minuscule number of us will be granted the realization of that fond hope. Such a devoutly wished-for consummation would demand a unique combination of nature, nurture, and luck given only to supremely rare individuals, who might be called outliers on the graph of human capability.

But as distinctively bestowed as such people may be—as remote as is the possibility that any of us will at a late stage of life be able to do the kinds of things they accomplish daily—there is yet a great deal to be learned by contemplating the examples they set. A great deal can be learned also by meditating on the ways in which personal philosophy can take maximal advantage of constitutional endowment, by meditating on the ways in which some individuals can forge a fusion of mind and body so remarkable that to be in its presence is to experience a surpassing awe for the potentialities of our species. Though perhaps in lesser ways and for a lesser time, the rest of us may learn much that is useful in the lessons these individuals' lives can teach. And who knows? There may be rare fortunate ones among us who, in later years, will look back and be able to say that we have survived to live life's final phase as fully as they have.

Such an exemplar of vibrant longevity is Dr. Michael De-Bakey. To appreciate what Dr. DeBakey has become in his late nineties requires an understanding of what he has been throughout his life, of which his present moment is only a smooth continuation. What follows here can encompass only the highlights of a remarkable career. Though seemingly a list, it is in fact an honor roll of contributions unmatched in the archive of twentieth-century medical science.

In 1931, while still a medical student at Tulane, twenty-two-year-old Michael DeBakey invented an ingenious roller pump for the propulsion of blood through flexible tubing. Though originally designed for use in circulation research being done by one of his teachers, the pump would twenty years later find a much more valuable application as the crucial component that enabled the development of the heart-lung machine for cardiac surgery.

As director of the Surgical Consultant Division of the Office of the Surgeon General during World War II, Colonel DeBakey made recommendations in several areas that led to major innovations in medical care and education, among them the development of mobile army surgical hospitals (the so-called MASH units) and the founding of the National Library of Medicine. He was also instrumental in organizing the structure that evolved into the Veterans Administration hospital system. In 1948, while in the midst of a burgeoning clinical and research career at Tulane, he was appointed chairman of surgery at Baylor University and began the process that built a world-famous center of innovation and patient care from the rudiments of a struggling medical school with neither an affiliated hospital nor a residency training program. Among his contributions in the next five years was the introduction of the Dacron artificial artery for reconstruction of damaged vessels. He was a pioneer—*the* pioneer, in fact—in surgery for aneurysms in the chest and abdomen, as well as in the treatment of the occlusions in the carotid artery to the brain that commonly cause strokes. He performed the first successful coronary artery bypass graft in 1964, of which thousands are now being done daily in hospitals throughout the world. So many are DeBakey's contributions and so prolific has he been in describing them in the pages of the scientific and clinical literature that the entire evolution of cardiovascular surgery is documented in his approximately sixteen hundred publications—and more are in process as these pages are being written. For these achievements and others, DeBakey was recognized for some four decades as the leading cardiovascular surgeon in the world.

In addition to technological achievements such as these, he has been a sought-after consultant to the government of the United States and many other countries, being frequently called upon to make major health policy recommendations as well as to provide surgical consultation and operative care to more than a few world leaders. Such missions have taken him to the former Soviet Union, for example, almost thirty times. *The American Journal of Cardiology* has hailed him as "the [twentieth] century's most influential international and national medical statesman," and the list of honors and titles awarded him by foreign governments and academic institutions goes on for page after page.

In the midst of all this, DeBakey was maintaining a perfectly huge surgical practice, eventually numbering some 60,000 operated patients, of whom he has long-term follow-up studies of 95 percent. Because of his reputation as a surgeon of remarkable dexterity and judgment, the well-worn path to his OR has been trod by the famous and humble of all sorts, from leaders of governments and celebrities of screen and popular entertainment to the many patients referred from the free clinics of Houston.

In the process of building the Baylor College of Medicine to its present eminence, DeBakey not only has been its surgical chairman, but has somehow found the time and energy to be its dean from 1969 to 1979, its chancellor from 1979 to 1996, and indubitably its guiding light throughout his long tenure in that place. And the school's reliance on his advice has hardly ended: During the visit I made to Houston in June 2005, the university's president came to consult with him over some particularly thorny administrative problem. In those precincts, he remains indispensable.

DeBakey has been the guardian spirit and the primary fund-raiser (and the prodigious personal donor of hundreds of millions of dollars), as well as the foremost teacher, clinician, and administrator of Baylor's medical center. The institution's entire intellectual and physical structure—not to mention its pulsing vitality—is the result of his leadership. To stand surrounded by the school's many acres of ultramodern and world-renowned medical buildings—into which some 60,000 staff members and employees enter each day—is to stand at the epicenter of DeBakey's career.

He operated until the age of ninety, during the final years working together with his former pupil Dr. George Noon. He eventually stopped, as he later told me, "Because there were so many other things that needed to be done." Patient evaluation and postoperative care consume a great deal of time, entailing a constant responsibility that was taking valuable hours and energy more effectively spent in his long-term follow-up studies, his laboratory research developing a cardiac assist device, and his ongoing travels as consultant to so many organizations and governments.

DeBakey and I became acquainted in 1998, when we spent a morning together before participating in a medical press conference in New York City. Since then, we have kept in touch by exchanging an occasional letter and sending each other recent articles we have written. As my thoughts began to turn increasingly toward consideration of the obstacles and opportunities presented by growing older, I from time to time thought about him and wondered at all he was continuing to accomplish. Finally, I decided to approach him as a surgeon should: directly.

I wrote to Dr. DeBakey in the spring of 2005 when he was ninety-six years old, and said that I wanted to visit him in Houston. His open and welcoming response was consistent with my previous experience of him, and within a few weeks I found myself, early on a still-sunny Sunday evening, waiting for him to pick me up outside the entrance to the hotel that is part of the huge medical complex at Baylor.

As I waited for my host to arrive, I let my gaze wander over the vast panorama of buildings that make up the Texas Medical Center. At least three times the size of my own medical complex in New Haven, everything there is in one form or another the product of DeBakey's leadership. His signature is figuratively stamped on the entire expanse of the place. Standing there, I could not help reflecting on the comment made by the son of London's great architect, Sir Christopher Wren (also a physician), shortly after the famous man's death at the age of ninety-one, in 1723. When asked where his father's monument would be, the son is said to have waved his arm as though to encompass the entire city, and said, "You have only to look around you to see it." In its Latin form— *Si monumentum requiris, circumspice*—those words would soon thereafter be inscribed in Wren's most renowned building, St. Paul's Cathedral. And thus it is with Baylor and Michael DeBakey.

From the hotel, we motored ("motored" is the only word to use when one is a Sunday passenger in a small Porsche sports coupe being driven by an internationally acclaimed multimillionaire heart surgeon) to the DeBakey home less than ten minutes away from the medical complex, where he has lived for some five decades. DeBakey's first wife, Diana, died suddenly of a heart attack in her early fifties, and he has been married for thirty years to the former Katrin Fehlhaber, who was a successful German film actress when he first met her at Jack Benny's eightieth birthday party, held at the home of Frank Sinatra, with whom DeBakey was staying while on a brief working visit to California. I mention these celebrity-soaked details to give some idea of the variegated shades, colors, and experiences in this singular man's adventure-filled life, in which moments with crowned heads, movie stars, and political eminences periodically punctuate the otherwise ceaseless intensity of clinical work, research, and the administration of a topflight academic institution to which he continues to devote his unflagging efforts after sixty years.

In her mid-fifties, Katrin DeBakey is one of those eternally vital women whose wholesome blond beauty is only enhanced by the passage of years. Her guests on that evening were a Lebanese-born cardiologist and his wife, with whom the dinner conversation moved easily across a variety of topics, in each of which our host revealed himself to be authoritative and remarkably well read. Not being accustomed to finding myself in the presence of surgeons with so many eclectic interests, and hardly expecting this one—especially considering the feverish pace of his professional life, abated only somewhat even at ninety-six—to be as deeply informed on such a wide range of subjects as he proved to be (not only during that evening, but throughout our subsequent time together), I sat in barely suppressed astonishment at the breadth of his knowledge of so many things. He demonstrated his familiarity with various examples of literature and poetry; the origins and theology of Islam and Christianity; the historical periods of the Reformation, the Renaissance, and the Industrial Revolution; aspects of the history of science; the eighteenth-century background to American democracy—to mention only the most prominent topics to which the evening's host responded or turned his and our attention.

As we stood near the door during that deliberately pro-longed point at the end of the evening when guests know they should leave but don't really want to, Katrin DeBakey re-sponded to something I had earlier said about seeking the basis of her husband's astounding vitality. I had spoken of its ingredients being his constitution (here read as genetic pre-disposition) plus what I called "something else," the nature of which I hoped to explore during my time in Houston. To her, the "something else" was hardly a mystery. "It's love," she said as if it were the most obvious thing in the world. "We live with love. My husband is surrounded by the love of his patients."

That response was not what I had expected. To me, a surgeon who had grown up professionally in the 1950s and '60s—a time when the streaking meteor of Michael DeBakey's career was rising ever upward—the gentle and selfless impli-cations brought to mind by thoughts of love were hardly those I associated with his name. His reputation was quite the opposite. This most talked-about surgeon of my era was said to be so single-mindedly dedicated to his craft that personal feeling fell—more than fell, was thrown—to the wayside. He could be cold and distant to his associates, it was said, and re-lentlessly demanding. He functioned at the epicenter of a tor-nado of activity that consumed every bit of the available energy in its whirling force field, and left bystanders agape at the power being generated by its forward motion. Where does love fit into such an image? How could it have figured as the "something else" of his longevity? Love coming from oth-ers has meaning only in proportion to its reflection in the love felt for them. It is thus a two-way street: If either direction is left untraveled, both are impassible.

Love and the kind of unremitting work to which DeBakey had devoted his career would seem at opposite poles, and yet, more than one thinker has linked them. Of course, apparent polar opposites are often found to be intimately connected one to the other. *Lieben und arbeiten* was virtually a motto for Sigmund Freud: To love and to work, he famously said, are the two keys to all that give life its meaning. Work is in itself a kind of love, we were told by DeBakey's fellow Lebanese American, the philosophic poet Kahlil Gibran, when he wrote, "Work is love made visible." When work is approached with love, he was saying, love can be its greatest reward.

Despite my skepticism, then, love would, in fact, prove to be the underlying theme in much of what DeBakey and I talked about during the subsequent day and a half of our discussions: love in its relationship to work, love as a gift given and gotten, love in all of its forms and manifestations. It would become clear that, just as DeBakey is consumed by his dedication to work, he is just as consumed by his dedication to his patients, each as a distinctive individual. His is no abstracted devotion to labor for its own sake. His labors are intertwined with a commitment to others.

DeBakey's research, for example, has not been done in emotion-free laboratories of basic science. The foundation and intent of his research are clinical, a word whose origin tells the origin of his determination in its pursuit, and in its own way bespeaks a kind of love. "Clinical" derives from the Greek noun *klinē,* or "bed," and therefore refers to a patient lying down, to a person and not some abstract object. That patient's welfare is the accelerant of the research, and such a fact alone gives the work a sense of personal urgency. Every bit of DeBakey's research and his labors in the operating rooms and clinics of Houston and elsewhere has been intended to benefit specific people for whom he has taken on responsibility. Though his contributions have been applied by others to the care of hundreds of thousands of men, women, and children, the incentive propelling the research arises from the needs of those individuals who, one at a time, have entrusted themselves to him alone. In treating each of them with the caring devotion of a dedicated physician, he has inspired the love of which his wife speaks. Love has been the warp, and work has been the woof, in the fabric of DeBakey's life and, as would become clear during our discussions, in the fabric of his longevity as well.

DeBakey's notion of work is not work alone but work driven by a sense of purpose so strong that it bears him forth as though on its wings. With that sense of purpose has evolved a sense of realism about what can be achieved, especially as age approaches and horizons must inevitably be drawn inward. To draw them closer in ways that make sense is to have found a wisdom about goals, priorities, changing abilities, and altered self-perceptions, which in itself requires that a certain serenity be found. Not unexpectedly, serenity, too, emerged as a theme of DeBakey's longevity. He has sought it in an unstructured religious faith that is his alone, which imparts not only serenity but a kind of mystical certainty of his relationship with a personal God and with all of humanity.

Though Katrin DeBakey's response to my question about the "something else" was not at all what I had anticipated, its meaning became more clear as I spoke with her husband during the next two days, much of which we spent huddled together at one end of a long table in the conference room that is part of his suite of offices. For all of his clinical, academic, and governmental achievements, I gradually came to see—both from his direct statements and by listening for it between the lines when he was discussing his longevity—that beyond all else, the factor that has given greatest meaning to this unexpectedly sensitive man's career is his ability to bring hope to the tens of thousands of individual men and women for whom he has cared. As he would early on the next morning tell me, "The gratification comes from the feeling that you've done something important for people. Life, after all, is the greatest thing we have, and doctors are in a unique position to maintain it, to save it, to give it."

Though speaking specifically of the unique position of physicians in their ability to maintain, save, or give life, De-Bakey was saying far more than he may have consciously thought. Doctors are indeed in a unique position for achieving this kind of gratification, but it struck me that there are wide-ranging implications in what he was describing, beyond sustaining physical health alone, or even life. As our discussions proceeded, I came to conclude that he was more generally referring to the broad range of interrelationships between individual people in which one can feel that he or she is doing something for another, whether it be a tangible thing like medical care and life, or primarily what might be called the emotional or spiritual, such as giving comfort and support, or encouraging the development of young people. What counts here is the giving, specifically the giving of one's abilities and consequently the giving of part of oneself to another. Simply put, the overall concept is the habit of living to ease the lives of one's fellows.

The dividends of such a life can come to each of us, in an awareness of having contributed something of value. The dividends of such a life come in an awareness of the climate of good that our own actions have fostered. The dividends of such a life come in an awareness of all that we represent to those who benefit from our time on this earth. The dividends of such a life come in an awareness of being appreciated and even cherished in return. And that is a form of love, which is the greatest dividend of all.

In such ways, the literal giving of health is revealed to be only one of the possible manifestations of the figurative. To put it another way, if "health" is defined, as it most properly is, as a state of well-being—whether physical, emotional, or spiritual—then it is within the province and capability of each of us to provide it for others. To give sustenance to another is the highest gift, both to him or her and to ourselves, that any of us can imagine. One hardly need be a doctor in order to do the giving. "The gratification comes from the feeling that you've done something for people."

Most of us know these kinds of things, though they have been robbed of a great deal of meaning because they have become the stuff of too much ponderous pap delivered from pulpits, the pages of maxim-filled hortatory literature, and the self-satisfied lips of an occasional latter-day Polonius. But in spite of the windy pontifications in which these ideas are sometimes expressed, mindfulness of them is inherent in human perception, though they are often ignored, forgotten, buried, or simply dismissed as the staggeringly banal pronouncements of would-be sages. But when expounded as the way of life of a man of DeBakey's worldly experience and philosophic gravitas, and—of perhaps equal significance—when brought forth as a strategy for long and useful living, the reminders for us to be of benefit to others are imbued with a power well beyond the turgid moralisms in which they are often couched. Examples of the truth of giving to others abound in everyone's life story, but I will here interrupt my DeBakey narrative to describe one to which I have been witness, as follows.

After recovering from a long and perilous illness about forty years ago, the then chaplain of Yale University, Reverend William Sloane Coffin, said a few words to me that changed my perception of the relationship between doctors and patients—indeed, the relationship between those who give and those who must receive, whether in respect to healing or in any other form. Having spent many weeks being treated on an acute care division of a busy university hospital, Coffin one day shortly before discharge made an observation about what he had seen: "We patients," he told me, "do more for you doctors than you do for us." By this he meant that the gratification of being able to help others is an abundance of reward rarely considered in the calculus of healing, or of any other form of giving of ourselves. Men and women who devote themselves to doing for others live enveloped in the nourishing aura of appreciativeness that oxygenates self-confidence and motivation. We are told in the Book of Acts that it is more blessed to give than to receive, and that ancient maxim has a lot to say for itself. Physicians and all manner of men and women actuated by the will to do good may not be consciously aware of it, but in their very giving they are blessed by those who receive. Seeing oneself reflected in the grateful eyes of a fellow human being to whom one has brought sustenance is surely among the most enriching of self-perceptions. It is in the very real sense a bountiful gift, one that must surely manifest itself not only in emotional but in physiological ways as well. That the encouragement of service to others is often expressed in flatulent aphorisms does not in any way lessen the worth of this service, and certainly does not diminish its value in relation to a long and satisfying life. It is not my purpose here to write a tract on saintliness as a path to longevity, or moral rectitude as a geriatric tonic. I am merely trying to focus on the ways that we may make the most of our final phase of life, and to extend it if we can.

And, of course, it is never too late. The getting and spending, the clawing rivalries, the need to prove ourselves to ourselves, the pragmatic drive to "succeed"—which so often motivate decision-making in earlier decades—are susceptible to softening as we reach our late-middle years, and continue to lessen their influence on our thinking as the decades pass. In these ways, the word "maturity" reassumes the meaning it had before the AARP and the pop psychologists of aging appropriated it for the purposes of feel-good. Of all the beneficences granted us by the evolving emotional changes that begin to make themselves manifest as we reach perhaps our early fifties, this maturity must surely be among the most valuable, both to those around us and to ourselves. Some of us are later than others in this kind of growing, and a few will never attain it. For many, it requires conscious effort to realize that it can be reached and to bring it to fullness. But in the ripening process of becoming ever more mature, far more of us than might be thought are increasingly able to leave off the shadowboxing of striving careerism, and emerge to a vision of ourselves that was unattainable at an earlier time. Done right, it most properly begins in middle life.

The fundamental notion of beneficent interactions between individuals emerged in many stated and unstated ways as DeBakey's musings traveled far and wide over the landscape of the "something else" that enables one person and not another to continue to function at a very high level—well beyond the age at which such high-level functioning is expected. But for a moment, it is necessary to return to that other factor, without which the "something else" cannot as effectively come into play. Even vast emotional rewards can affect longevity only up to a point if the physical fiber—so much of which comes with our genes—is wanting. Ourselves are held back without our stars, to turn Cassius's admonition to Brutus on its head. All the "something else" in the world avails only so much when the constitution lacks, whether that constitution's ingredients are inherited or have been maximized by good fortune and life's experiences. And here, DeBakey enters the race with that combination of DNA, resistance to rust, and good luck that forms the basis for the something else. His father died at ninety; his mother at almost eighty of malignancy; three of his four siblings are still alive in their nineties; the other, a sister, died of cancer in her eighties; he has never suffered a major illness or accident; save for his first wife's premature death, his life has been free of tragedy or the debilitating unhappiness inflicted by the sorts of externals over which one has no control.

The age of DeBakey's siblings is of particular interest in view of the findings of the New England Centenarian Study, which to no one's surprise found that centenarians are four times more likely than others to have a sibling who lived beyond the age of ninety. But even this is not in itself indubitable evidence that DeBakey's long living is heavily indebted to heredity. As those who did the study would be the first to point

out, members of the same family share more than DNA—they
tend to have similar values, and they tend to share such characteristics as eating habits and attitudes toward exercise and
intellectual stimulation.

And then there is the matter of DeBakey's diet. Altogether,
we shared four meals during my visit, which included two
dinners and two lunches. As he always does, my host ate very
little, and he does not hesitate to point out that he thinks this
may be a contributing factor to his longevity and to his generally robust health. He bases his opinion on a series of experimental studies indicating substantial prolongation of the
lives of laboratory animals fed a diet very low in calories. As
I observed DeBakey at each meal, I would estimate that the
volume of food he ate was about half mine, or less. At dinner
on our second evening, he ordered a dish of pasta and ate
one-third of it, which he told me is his usual habit.

And thus, DeBakey has been mightily equipped by nature,
circumstance, and choice with qualities necessary for what
the seventeenth-century physician-philosopher Sir Thomas
Browne in his *Hydriotaphia* called "the long habit of living."
At ninety-six, DeBakey looked no older than seventy. Though
he has not done a whit of fitness exercise since his youth, his
five feet ten inches are lean and wiry at 150 pounds. To
demonstrate his muscle tone, he at one point pulled up the
sleeve of his lab coat and contracted a biceps that projected
like a tennis ball from his upper arm, and with the same
firmness.

Though there can be no doubt that DeBakey has in such
benisons of fate or good fortune been better provisioned than
most of us, that cannot alone explain what he is today, in the
second half of his tenth decade. There has to be far more, and

the more must certainly reveal patterns as useful to everyone as the concept of service to others. Of what, in fact, does the rest of the "something else" consist?

Here is Michael DeBakey explaining it to me, and perhaps, by giving it a literal articulation, explaining it to himself as well:

> It is this aspect of seeking knowledge, and, to use an even more direct word, curiosity. Curiosity and the seeking of knowledge is a transcendent life force—almost, you might say, spiritual. It has a driven character to it. It drives you intellectually and, to an extent, physiologically. The brain influences the body in ways we don't know about.

Here DeBakey is describing what might be called a forward momentum created by the very process of seeking knowledge. As I thought about this notion, both while De-Bakey was speaking and while ruminating on it later, it became increasingly clear that these few sentences elucidate not only a key factor in his continuing productivity, but also a clue to the success of his entire career. He goes to bed each night, he told me at one point, looking forward to the morning so that he can do those things he was unable to accomplish on that day. The propulsive momentum of the thing was evident in his description: work to be done, plans to be made, places to go, things to learn—ever new challenges to be taken up. Were I asked to put a name to it all, I would call it the anticipation of the interesting.

Anticipation would seem to be just the right term, because it incorporates the notion of eagerly looking forward to promised intellectual stimulation whose taste can already be almost felt. This urgency of expectance would seem to be the essence of the thing about which DeBakey was speaking. When he uses the word "driven," the force and magnitude of the anticipation are exactly what he means. He is driven by the imagined taste of coming pleasure. His mind already senses its flavor because he has known it all his life. Michel de Montaigne wrote about such things: "In every pleasure known to man the very pursuit of it is pleasurable. The undertaking savours of the quality of the object it has in view; it effectively constitutes a large proportion of it and is cosubstantial with it."

The notion of the imminence of immanent pleasure extrapolates to so many other circumstances, for so many other people. Like beneficence, it is available to all of us. And also like beneficence, it may be an acquired taste, taking hold of us or being deliberately sought not until middle or later years as more time is available and opportunities increase—or perhaps as the energy of career and striving transform themselves imperceptibly into the energy of learning and creativity for their own sakes. For DeBakey, such imminence is the foretaste of new knowledge and the modified continuation of a career. For others, it may be in the anticipated pleasure of working in a blossoming garden; creating an artistic piece of pottery or woodworking; improving a game of golf; seeing old friends; traveling to new places; learning to play a musical instrument or studying a foreign language; finding joy in children's children; or some combination of all of these and similar enjoyments. In the house of anticipation there are many mansions, each distinctive to the life of the man or woman who finds it. Some pleasurable pursuits arise from the edifice of a career and long-standing interests, as do DeBakey's. Some are entirely new discoveries. Either way, these pursuits provide the promise of oncoming pleasure that can be the power source of a vitality that propels us forward. They are the drive of which DeBakey speaks. Each of these pursuits is a form of creativity, and each of them can—and should—be discovered long before we begin sliding into old age.

But the propulsions that can drive later life come with necessary caveats that need to be observed. And in DeBakey's advice about such things, we once again encounter the warning that one must look down even while looking up:

> When there are things to be done, they must be done whether you're ninety-six or fifty-six. Those are just numbers. But I think that conceptually it's important as you age to recognize some of the limitations that age produces. But once you've recognized them, then you are aware of those limitations and this allows you to be flexible within them.

What is being said here is that knowing one's limitations and learning to function within them allows the avoidance of the unmanageable. By doing this, it becomes possible to work most effectively in order to achieve chosen aims, without dispersing energy on what can no longer be achieved and then being forced to deal with the thwarting disappointment that necessarily follows. In an earlier chapter, this was described as letting our horizons come closer, and confining our plans to the realistic.

> While I know what my limitations are, I also know that by those limitations and by my realizing what they are

and working within them, I avoid allowing them to interfere with what I want to do. It doesn't in any way restrict my intellectual capabilities.

By doing that, you see, you also avoid the frustration. This is important to do, in order to maintain the serenity that can affect your life and whatever you're going to do. Frustration is an enemy in your life. It can be one of the very important negative factors upon your health and your life. So you must deal with it. Otherwise it harms you—it's harmful to be frustrated too long, and I've learned from my early experience to deal with it and with anger in so many ways—even spiritually sometimes. The same is true with anger. Anger is in some respects a form of frustration. These are things you have to learn how to handle, and as you grow older they become more important, because age also tends to make things much less flexible than they were in your youth. One of the major advantages of youth is its greater flexibility, both mentally and physically. You can substitute for that as you grow older, with what I call wisdom.

Until this point, DeBakey had been speaking of attitudes that serve to sustain intellectual and physical vigor, and, indeed, such matters formed the substance of our discussion. But of equal importance is to avoid patterns of thinking that have a negative effect on powers that might remain intact were they not actively lessened by counterproductive or harmful ways of thinking.

One of the problems of aging is that the mind is ahead of the body. I've noted that some people—some of my colleagues, in fact—have allowed their bodies to deteriorate because they perceive themselves to be old. In other words, they have become impressed with the fact that they are old in years, and therefore respond by *being* old—and I'm using "old" in the sense of true physical deterioration. Of course, there *is* a certain amount of that, which does occur with age. Those people who have been blessed with a physical constitution that has maintained intellectual fervor, intellectual vigor, have to come to a certain, you might say, accommodation with the physical limitations that they are no longer able to control.

And so, DeBakey is reiterating, once we understand our limitations and accept them, we can learn to work within them. This is the form of wisdom of which he is here speaking; this is the form of wisdom that brings the serenity that allows us to cope with frustration and anger. Obviously, all of this is circular, with each component feeding back into the others, strengthening them even as it gains strength from them.

I did very little talking as we discussed these matters—there was no need for it. I was communing with a man who was not merely responding to questions put to him, but was, in fact, explicating convictions to which he had quite obviously given a great deal of thought over many years. The words came easily, because they were the expression of long-evolving certainties.

I wanted to know about the role played by faith in DeBakey's thinking, not only faith's involvement in fortune, but also the ways in which faith contributes to the serenity on which he places so much emphasis.

DeBakey was brought up in the Greek Orthodox church of

his immigrant Lebanese parents, "in a religious atmosphere," as he puts it. He has tasted of other faiths, and clearly has a wide knowledge of religious forms and practices. But his beliefs are nowadays not restricted to the tenets of an organized church; they are his alone, though he describes their most personal manifestations in terms that many other men and women might recognize as being similar to their own.

> I have been secure in the knowledge that I have had a relationship with my God, and that he was going to take care of me. My childhood experience in my parents' religion has changed in what I call having matured. I don't think of faith any longer as a child does, and yet I have retained that spiritual relationship with a God that I had as a child—because it gives me a feeling of serenity to do so. I'm not a regular churchgoer, but there again, that's part of the maturity I'm talking about. I don't think I need to go to church. People used to ask me in interviews what church I go to and I'd say, "Yes, I'm in church right now." I'm in church wherever I am. I'm in church at home, I'm in church here. My relationship with God is a personal one.

Thoughts of faith led to questions about belief in afterlife.

> I don't know about that, and I'm not concerned about it. Right now I *am* in a life. I'm secure in my relationship with my God, and I don't need to worry about an afterlife and don't need to have a sense of insecurity about what's going to happen to me. To me, that is part, again, of what I mean by maturity.

The maturity seems to go even further than DeBakey is prepared to say. I could not resist pondering just how much this most self-reliant of men actually does expect from his God. I may have found the answer in a brief article he published only four months before my visit, in the academic journal *Surgery*, revealingly entitled "Kismet or Assiduity?" The article appeared as part of a series in which distinguished contributors are asked to write brief narratives of personal history or surgical lore. In it, DeBakey tells of taking the oral examination of the American Board of Surgery in 1938, and being asked to evaluate a forty-year-old man ten days post-appendectomy, who had developed fever, right-sided abdominal pain, and an elevated white blood cell count. The young candidate correctly diagnosed an abscess under the diaphragm, a conclusion aided by DeBakey's having recently published a paper on the subject that had, by seemingly lucky coincidence, been read by one of his two examiners, Dr. Fred Rankin. (To this day, that paper is considered a classic description of the problem.) When a few years later Colonel Rankin heard about DeBakey's army enlistment shortly after the attack on Pearl Harbor, he arranged for the new recruit to be assigned to the Surgical Consultant Division in the Office of the Surgeon General, of which Rankin was the head. It was there that DeBakey made his important contributions to the origins of the MASH units, the National Library of Medicine, and the system of veterans hospitals described earlier. In time, he succeeded Dr. Rankin as head of the division.

In the final paragraph of "Kismet or Assiduity?" DeBakey muses over whether it was destiny or his own hard work that conspired to make his good fortune. "In classical literature," he writes, "fate was sometimes defined as ineluctably predestined," and then he goes on to quote the famous *Rubaiyat* verse about the immutability of words written by the Moving Finger. But in the end, the ninety-six-year-old author of the article comes down solidly in favor of hard work, concluding his piece with a stanza from Longfellow's "A Psalm of Life."

> *Let us, then, be up and doing,*
> *With a heart for any fate;*
> *Still achieving, still pursuing,*
> *Learn to labor and to wait.*

Religious belief, kismet, and enviable DNA notwithstanding, there seems little doubt that Michael DeBakey has made his own psalm of life. Its theme is assiduity.

Having spoken of the past, the present, and the afterlife, I broached the question of DeBakey's future years. What sort of hopes does a ninety-six-year-old man have for the time left to him? Though blessed with constitution and having found that "something else" we had been delving into, he was nevertheless ninety-six, and though it is "just a number," nothing can change it. There are, after all, limits to how far even his prodigious endowments and philosophy can take him. Has he set goals for his remaining days?

I don't dwell on it, and so as a consequence I don't come to a final schedule. Philosophically, I suppose, the basic reason for that is that I don't want to *make* a schedule. If I do that, it makes me dwell on the schedule and that makes me dwell on its termination.

I've long accepted the fact of my own death. I'm ready whenever it comes, in the sense that I know I can't stop it.

But I don't dwell on it. As long as I feel physically and mentally like I feel now, and stay asymptomatic and have a schedule of things that need to be done, I don't think about whether or not I'm going to be alive to do them. So, knowing that sooner or later *something* is going to happen to me, I just go ahead. When I get on a plane, for example, I'm absolutely sure I'll arrive to where I'm going.

"I'm absolutely sure I'll arrive to where I'm going." The sentence echoes in my mind. I've listened to it over and over, rising up from the tape that recorded it. It seems to encompass Michael DeBakey's reflections on the grace and rewards of aging.

Kismet, assiduity, and every other factor that has made Michael DeBakey the man that he is—all of them came to a focus on February 9, 2006, eight months after my visit to Houston, when a team composed of several generations of surgeons who had trained under his supervision operated on him for a life-threatening thoracic aneurysm, an acute disruption of the largest blood vessel in the body a few inches beyond its origin in the heart. The operation they performed on their chief, which is one of the most hazardous and complex in all surgery, was an updated modification of the one DeBakey had introduced in February 1954. The equipment and technology that made it possible were all the result of his originality and inventiveness.

Only a few years earlier, a team of surgeons from the DeBakey Department of Surgery at Baylor had published a paper in the *Journal of Vascular Surgery* entitled "Emergency

Surgery for Thoracoabdominal Aortic Aneurysms with Acute Presentation," reporting on 112 patients operated upon between 1986 and 1998, with a mortality of 17 percent, a remarkably low figure for such a lethal condition. But perhaps even more remarkable than such outstanding results was their finding that "age did not influence survival rate." The mean age of the patients in the series was seventy, plus or minus eight years. On the day of his operation, Michael DeBakey was ninety-seven.

DeBakey not only survived, but applied his assiduity to a vigorous program of physical rehabilitation that might have cowed many a younger man. In September 2006, a few days after his ninety-eighth birthday, and shortly before he flew to New York for a research awards luncheon, I received a letter from him in which he wrote, "I am doing very well and hope to have the pleasure of seeing you again sometime soon."

FOUR

MAKING CHOICES

The unexamined life is not worth living.
—Plato, *Apology of Socrates,* ca 400 BCE

If you look at a problem long enough, you can see the part you play in it.
—Miriam Fox Gabler, *Ozarks Senior Living,* 2005

The name of Miriam Fox Gabler will not be remembered half a dozen decades from now. Her son and daughter—both adopted—are in their late forties and childless; her long line of DNA will die with her final breath. She will leave no personal legacy to any generations of descendants. Almost certainly, no one will think about her late in this century, to remember the deeds she did and the lessons she taught. After a time, all memory of her will disappear. It will be as though she had never lived.

The name of Plato, on the other hand, and the words he recorded as those of Socrates will echo through the culture of civilization as long as humankind survives. Plato could not have known there would be a Miriam Gabler. To Miriam Gabler, Plato is a barely perceived figure from the classical past, a vaguely known and ancient philosopher with whose thoughts she is unfamiliar. She has never read his aphorism quoted above, nor any other sentences he wrote.

But were Miriam Gabler ever to see those words, she would surely know what to make of them, as they have meaning for her own life. She would understand them to express her conviction that it is incumbent on those who have achieved a good measure of contentment in their lives to conjure with themselves about its sources and its continuity, and about the choices that might so easily have led to its opposite. She is not content to be content without context: Like Plato, Miriam Gabler believes that earnest examining of one's life opens the way to conscious decisions to improve it, and thereby adds to its value and its rewards.

And so, Miriam studies the reasons for her contentment. She has made herself aware not only of the portion of it that seems to have been dealt her by chance and circumstance, but of the part as well that she has been able to "play in it." And in at least this way, Plato and Miriam Gabler—an immortal and a woman destined to be forgotten—walk together.

I met Miriam in the final days of 2005, a scant three weeks after the death of her husband. He had a decade earlier first developed the confusion that proved to be the earliest indication of Alzheimer's disease—so gradual in manifesting its ul-

timate destructive effects that it could not be diagnosed until
five years later, in 2000. Progression was more rapid after
that time, and by September 2001 he had to be admitted to a
nursing home. Miriam spent hours of every day with Don, as
his ability to know or even recognize the world around him
lessened with each passing week. It was a terrible time for her,
a time of sadness beyond measure—and of desperate yearning for the love she had found so late in life and was now
losing.

Miriam's first marriage, in 1947 to Frank Marshall when
she was twenty-one, had been difficult almost from the start.
Because she underwent a hysterectomy at twenty-three for a
fibroid uterus, the couple adopted two children, Mark and
Debby. The marriage became more strained and distant as
time wore on, and a divorce was agreed upon in 1970, when
Miriam was forty-four. After eleven years of bringing up her
children as a single mother, she met an electrician named Don
Gabler, and something in her came to life again. It was of no
consequence to either of them that she was six years his senior. "Together we found everything that was missing in our
first marriages."

After Miriam and Don married in 1989, their joy in each
other only continued to increase. "I was sixty-two at the time
of our wedding, a no-nonsense woman with graying hair.
He was fifty-six, youthfully handsome and a terribly sweet
guy." Even long after Don began to experience the disturbing
episodes that appeared at first to be only mild confusion, the
couple's happiness seemed assured. But after six years of gradual worsening and a trial of day care, Miriam finally agreed
to let her husband be admitted to a nursing facility near their
home in Mystic.

It was two years later that Miriam one day came to her moment of realization, a moment characteristic of her enduring ability to clarify issues, especially those involved in the series of misfortunes she had endured before meeting Don. In her usual contemplative way, she had been looking hard at her problem, and could now finally recognize the part she played in it. The culmination of that self-examining was the recognition of what had to be done. She recognized it so well, in fact, that she was able to clearly articulate her decision to herself and also to those who would later read about it in a brief article she wrote that very evening, for a monthly publication called *Ozarks Senior Living*. The date was January 12, 2003, the anniversary of her marriage to Don.

LONG OVERDUE

Today I made a choice. I could cry and be miserable because my husband is in a nursing home, or I could rejoice that on this day fourteen years ago, I became his wife.

Don is a victim of Alzheimer's. It has been a long grieving process. Today I chose to be thankful for the beautiful life we shared before he became ill. No one ever loved me as he did. I no longer believe love is blind. I believe love sees what nobody else can see.

He was a youthful forty-nine when we met—tall, dark and deliciously handsome. I was six years older, a no-nonsense woman intimidated by our age difference and captivated by his playfulness. In early January, 1989, surrounded by four of our six children, we were married.

A million times since that day, he stroked my wrinkled face and patted my silver hair.

"My gorgeous wife," he murmured, his bright eyes shining. We never tired of talking, sharing our most intimate thoughts. We laughed, danced, and thrilled to the ecstasies of renewed youth. Neither time nor progression of his disease can erase the beauty of our relationship.

This morning I baked an angel food cake, Don's favorite, and carried a slice with me when I visited him. I broke it into tiny pieces that he could manage. I hugged and kissed him, and told him it was a special day. He looked at me with faint recognition. "I love you," I said, proud of myself for not crying.

Driving home I acknowledged that it was indeed a special day. Not only did it commemorate fourteen years of marriage to a beautiful human being, but it was the day I received the grace to make a healthy choice . . . long overdue.

Miriam gave me a copy of the article as we sat talking in the living room of the small house she had shared with Don in Mystic, a Connecticut seaport town very near the Rhode Island state line. She lives on a quiet street of only four houses, called Misty View Avenue, so named, no doubt, on account of the thin fog that frequently rolls in from the nearby confluence of Long Island Sound and the Atlantic Ocean. It was late on the Friday afternoon before Christmas, and we were talking about her life.

At that time, I was about eight months into the study and writing that eventually became this book, and I was becoming intrigued by an issue too infrequently addressed in the literature on aging: How is the quest for so-called successful aging affected when it must be carried out in the face of a history and the aftereffects of life-threatening illness? It is all well and good for age sages to promote the virtues of optimism, creativity, and a healthy lifestyle, but how has the achieving of such goals been accomplished by men and women who have had to deal, for example, with cancer, stroke, or one of the many other stumbling blocks that all too often clutter the path toward the sixties and beyond? Do not such burdens thereafter weigh too heavily on the mind to allow any significant measure of the emotional serenity that is so necessary to a rewarding old age?

Over the previous month, I had been pondering the possible answers to such questions. It was clear that the obvious and expected was true, namely, that those men and women who were able to put their diseases into perspective and who had not allowed themselves to become emotionally crippled by them were most likely to go on to rewarding older age. In other words, the response to the physiological insult is more important than the insult itself. That part of the problem is self-evidently simple. But what determines any given individual's response, and what are the ingredients of such a response?

I would in time find that some of these successful men and women had significantly altered their perceptions of life and their values as a result of their sickness, while others had somehow been able to remain blithely untouched by it. But the quality uniting all who overcame such problems was that they had not allowed their determination to be derailed, whether they had integrated their experience into a changed philosophy of living or had treated the experience like a mere bump in the road, now passed and well behind them.

With all of this in mind, I was curious to know the details

of how such successful people had dealt with their setbacks. What might some of the factors be that determine whether having been seriously ill has a positive, a negative, or no effect on the ability to deal well with the aging process? How important are bonds of love and friendship—the support that comes from close relationships of trust? Does having a self-sufficient personality, for example, exclude the need for the devotion of, and for, others? What role does religion play? How do those who have overcome the burden of illness think about death and the possibility of an afterlife? And finally, in speaking to men and women who have overcome so much and gone on to rewarding years of older age, I wanted to know how they would wish to be remembered.

All of these questions were on my mind as Miriam Gabler and I sat talking together in the small living room of her comfortable little house on Misty View Avenue. Even our one distraction was of a piece with the unpretentious snugness of the atmosphere she had created in that place: the frequent nuzzling against my leg of Miriam's little beagle, Lucy, loving even a stranger and so certain of being loved in return that she expected to be stroked and petted by every visitor.

Miriam and I had pulled our chairs up to a small round table from atop which a soft shaded glow spread outward to supplement the declining light of the late December afternoon's setting sun. Bending just a bit forward toward each other as people do when absorbed in conversation, we could have been mistaken for two elderly friends come together for tea and a congenial chat. Everything about that room and the feeling it invoked in me, I soon came to realize, was the reflection of Miriam herself, and of the contentedness she has found in the everyday richness of her life.

I had come the sixty miles from New Haven because of a letter I had received the week before from a woman whose name was unfamiliar to me, Miriam Gabler, thanking me for the chapter on Alzheimer's disease in *How We Die*. Authors of expository books receive many such letters, and each is so interesting in its own way that I have answered almost all of those that have come to me over the years, and Mrs. Gabler's was no exception. But reflecting on her words a few days later in light of some of the questions I was then thinking about, I realized that she might be precisely the sort of person I had been wanting to meet.

It was clear from the letter that my correspondent had long since come to an acceptance of her husband's disease, but she wrote also of something else, and it piqued my interest: She had undergone surgery and irradiation therapy for ovarian cancer more than forty years earlier. The tone of the letter, the voice in which these potentially fragmenting events—her troubled marriage and the divorce, her cancer, her much-loved husband's decline into dementia and death—were recounted, reflected such a thoughtfully sober intelligence that it spoke of something beyond mere coping; it spoke of a certain knowing integration of the grim facts of sickness and great loss into the fabric of a life that not only had made peace with adversity but had gone beyond peace into the strength that familiarity with misfortune can sometimes bring.

It was while rereading the letter that "content," the word I later came to associate with Miriam Gabler, first entered my thoughts. At seventy-nine, she had quite obviously not been satisfied with becoming merely reconciled to her difficulties: She was content and even happy with her life; content and eager to have more of it exactly as it was; content and even determined to use her experience of adversity as a source of the wisdom that could continue to sustain her. She asked no more of life than was hers at that moment, which to her was satisfaction enough. All of this had come clear in the five brief but immensely revealing paragraphs of her letter. As I would learn when I met Miriam, she had long ago made a carefully deliberated decision—the first of many—not to let her life come undone.

Miriam Fox grew up in Norwich, Connecticut, the fourth of five children of Russian Jewish immigrants who owned a barely viable soda-delivery business. Encouraged by a doting father, she studied bookkeeping in high school and took a full-time job after graduation. Her conversion to Catholicism at the time of her marriage to Frank Marshall two years later predictably caused a furor in the family, leaving her mother with lifelong smoldering resentment. Her father, on the other hand, overcame his disappointment and was able to forgive his favorite child. Unlike many who convert for marriage, Miriam never took her new religion lightly, schooling herself and becoming as devout a Catholic as though she had been born to it.

Miriam and Frank were divorced eight years after her 1962 treatment for ovarian cancer. She went back to bookkeeping in order to support herself and the two children, but her health was never the same after the illness. The series of X-ray treatments that had helped cure her cancer brought its own problems, consisting of radiation damage sufficient to cause multiple bouts of intestinal obstruction over the years, and a tendency toward frequent loose stools, a problem that worsened after 1992 when at age sixty-six she was diagnosed with another cancer, this one of the large bowel. The required surgery excised the right side of the colon and a considerable length of the most involved portion of the small bowel that had been scarred and bound into dense adhesions by the previous operation and subsequent X-ray therapy. From then on, even more frequent stools continued to be a problem, necessitating great care in choice and preparation of foods.

As a result of the many years of constant bowel looseness and periodic obstruction, Miriam, at five feet four inches and one hundred pounds, is a very thin, slight woman, but only physically. There is nothing of debilitation about her. On the contrary, her determined visage, a clear and evenly modulated voice, and the direct gaze with which she regards me as we exchange greetings on my arrival and throughout our hours together give her the appearance of a petite and totally self-reliant matriarch accustomed to the give and take of an engaged life. There is an unmistakable tenacity about her, already apparent within our first moments of conversation.

Thanks to a meticulous caution with diet, Miriam is not at all malnourished. The caution consists of choosing foods well and of extreme attention to the details of preparation. But she so loves her kitchen that pains taken with cookery are hardly a burden for her. In fact, she thinks of cooking in much the same way as she does the other creative activities that bring her pleasure. What is a nuisance, though, is the problem of a cataract in her left eye, so dense that she needs to carry a magnifying glass when she goes shopping, in order to read the small print on labels. She cheerfully puts up with a disability she considers negligible, because both she and her ophthalmologist are reluctant to consider surgery.

Like so many other men and women in their late seventies,

Miriam takes several drugs to control an element of coronary disease and hypertension. And, of course, she has needed constant medications to keep her stools under reasonable control. Considering all that her body has been through over the past six decades, her total of five prescription drugs is no more than the average for someone her age.

Early in our conversation that afternoon, Miriam made it clear that her present contentment has not come about unplanned. Even before reaching middle age, the examination of a life not her own had led her to a deliberate decision to cultivate interests that would serve her well in later years. The life she examined was her mother's, a chronically dissatisfied woman who had never developed the independence or interests that might have brought some measure of enjoyment into an existence that gradually became more isolated and embittered toward the end of her life. "I resolved that I wouldn't let such a thing happen to me when I got older. I've realized recently that I may not have had the sense to plan my life, but I did plan my old age. I decided even in my late twenties that I wouldn't be like my mother. I'd find things I could be interested in, so that when I'm older, I'd have plenty to do."

The first of the "things" Miriam undertook was a writing course when she was thirty, done by correspondence with an organization called Writer's Digest. Since then, she has taken other such courses, at a nearby community college and elsewhere. An easy, articulate literary style attests to the courses' effect on her ability to transmit her thoughts in direct and absorbing sentences. Hers is a style influenced not only by years of attention to craftsmanship but also by her having acquired an associate degree in general studies at the same community college, when she was fifty-four. In fact, she embarked on a bachelor's program but "never got very far because Don came on the scene to distract me."

As she reached her later years, and particularly after the onset of Don's illness, Miriam increasingly turned to writing as a way to study and clarify her own thinking and sometimes to share it with others. Her real purpose was to explore her mind in words, as a way of understanding feelings and the circumstances in which she found herself. But she did submit some of her musings for publication, and has been very successful. As I've pored over some of the twenty-three articles she has published in a variety of periodicals—ranging from *The Providence Journal* to the magazine for the elderly called *Ozarks Senior Living,* produced in Springfield, Missouri— I've found myself thinking of Miriam's as a sensitive, insightful, and candid voice for so many older women, and perhaps men too, living alone, who find meaning in what some might deride as merely the humdrum details of their daily doings: braiding a rug, cooking, buying a cemetery plot, resolving a personal issue, reminiscing about a beloved father long gone. These are the topics of some of the pieces she has written over the decades, but more frequently in recent years.

Many of the "humdrum details" in Miriam's writing are centered on the few small rooms of the home that is so much the expression of herself that she seems as comfortably clothed in it as she does in the warm-toned slacks and blouse she is wearing during our conversation. This woman is so much of a piece with the envelopment she has created around herself that even a stranger feels embraced by it. "I love my home. I wake up here each morning and I'm happy that I have just one more day. I don't know what to do first. What I pray for is to remain in this house as long as I can take care of myself. I'm just so pleased to be here in this place of mine—writing, reading, quilting, braiding rugs, cooking. I love to cook. Here, let me show you a poem I treasure that spells it out for me." With this, Miriam gets up, goes to her small study, and brings back a copy of Alice Walker's "Grace."

Grace
Gives me a day
Too beautiful
I had thought
To stay indoors
& yet
Washing my dishes
Straightening
My shelves
Finally
Throwing out
The wilted
Onions
Shrunken garlic
Cloves
I discover
I am happy
To be inside looking out.
This, I think,
Is wealth.
Just this choosing
Of how
A beautiful day
Is spent.

For other reasons too, but particularly for her cherishing of this poem that conveys so much of the richness that Miriam has found in her daily life, the word "content" comes so readily to mind as my image of the entirety of her. There is a happiness in this image of Miriam, a happiness bespeaking an implicit inner assurance by which a world made small and safe is contemplated through the self-aware eye. Through such an eye Miriam sees the good within which it is possible to enfold oneself when horizons of ambition have been drawn close enough to encompass a sheltering surround of tranquility and familiar things. "To be inside looking out. / This, I think, / Is wealth."

"So many people seem to be unhappy," Miriam says, and a tone of impatience creeps into her voice. "They can't be satisfied; they can't solve anything. I can't waste my time with that sort of thing, and I can't waste time with people who don't nourish me." She is an active member of the local senior center, where she has taken several courses, including quilting and rug-braiding—and more writing. There is so much to do. "My days are so satisfying. I love this life of mine, and the big thing is to appreciate it. It was the experience with ovarian cancer that first had such an influence on me in that regard. It played a big part in teaching me that time is so precious, and so are people. And the intestinal cancer just added to that feeling." "Sweet are the uses of adversity," counseled the Bard. "Sermons in stones, and good in every thing." Miriam has used her adversity well.

Between the lines of all that she describes is a sense of the commitment to the areas in which she finds fulfillment. Miriam is not just a little old lady who sends brief articles off to magazines—she has made of herself a skilled writer who works hard at improving her craftsmanship, and at reaching into the depths of her mind and experience to find words and ways that might most clearly respond to her literary needs and the needs of her readers. The rug-braiding, the quilting, the cooking—all of these are arts to her, just as they are sources of contentment. "It's not enough to be busy. The busyness must have meaning." The very fact of her horizons' nearness magnifies the plenitude of all they encompass.

But to Miriam, the ineffable spirituality that she intuits even beyond those horizons has brought a kind of transcendence. "I want to serve God in some way," she tells me, and that way has been illumined for her by what she refers to as the "tremendous role that faith has played" in her life. She has been a devoted Catholic for more than half a century, and always very active in her parish. She still attends mass almost every week but no longer says the rosary or goes to confession. Though she loves worship and especially the music, her belief nowadays manifests itself less within the well-marked boundaries of Catholicism, and gradually has become defined in a far more personalized way, a way that remarkably enough takes account of a lingering sense of the Jewishness into which she was born. "I consider myself a Jewish Christian," she tells me, "and I have a precious relationship with my God." She prays often, largely in a nonformalized way that is hers alone. In a letter she later wrote to me, she says, "I believe as Martin Buber did, that God lives wherever man lets him. For that gift I have experienced the greatest sufferings and the greatest joys of my life."

Also nonformalized is Miriam's approach to her own death. Does she think about it, I ask her, and does she have any formed notions of what lies beyond? "I do think about it sometimes, but I'm not afraid of it. If I drop dead, be happy for me. It doesn't disturb me that I have no answers to what happens after death. The fact is that I'm too busy living to be worried about dying."

A great part of the being too busy is Miriam's relationships with the people around her, whether in the senior center, her church, or the community of Mystic. "Relationships is my middle name," she states emphatically, and her manner of saying those words conveys the enthusiasm with which she engages with people. But here, too, she does not spread herself widely or indiscriminately. Just as she needs others—including her son and daughter—to nurture her, she needs to nurture others. "I would like to be remembered as helping other people. I think life is difficult, and I can sometimes do or say things that make it easier for people who need what I can give." When Miriam says, "I thank God for my ability to deal with my life," there is no mistaking that "thank God" is an expression of religious belief and not merely the usual meaningless turn of phrase as most of us are inclined to use it. If anything has sustained Miriam Gabler through the times of being beset with so much, it is her unshakable trust that God has been guiding her life. "A belief in a higher power is a tremendous help, and the trust in God that you're living the life you were meant to live, and, God willing, you'll accept it. Trust is so important to me. Because I trust in God, I'm willing to accept whatever comes. I'm trying to be very realistic about where I am in life. I feel very grateful."

Miriam attributes her self-reliance to her reliance on faith, to a trust in God that seems inherent within her. Though she has long followed the Catholic rite, the source of her faith seems as independent of it as it is independent of the Judaism that first introduced her to belief. In one of the letters we exchanged after our meeting, she wrote, "I'd like you to know that at age nineteen I was engaged to a nice Jewish boy. When I suggested to him that we attend services, he laughed at me. I broke the engagement. At twenty-one I married Frank Marshall, getting 'hooked' when he said his religion was important to him. I learned much later that his relationship was with the Catholic Church. He had none with God."

I interpret "I'd like you to know" as meaning that the thing Miriam really wants me to know is that, to her, the basic trust is in God, and only secondarily in religious forms. I was struck by this partly because of a meeting I had had perhaps a month earlier, with a man totally free of faith in either God or religion, who in his own way is aging as successfully as Miriam is. But their relative positions on the spectrum of reliance on higher powers was only the tip of an iceberg of differences between them.

The most visible difference is physical. William G. "Pete" Barker is one of those elegantly tall (six feet one inch, and 175 pounds) and prosperous-looking executive types who are to be seen gracing the front pews of Episcopal churches every Sunday morning, along with their attractively wholesome wives and children, in such Connecticut towns as Greenwich, Darien, and New Canaan. While Pete *is* nominally Episcopalian and a retired executive, and he does live in Greenwich—and is, to fill in another bit of the picture, a loyal-to-the-point-of-fervent Dartmouth alumnus—he is in most other ways very much a species singularly his own. So far removed is he from ever being sighted in those patrician pews that he has to think a moment when I ask him his religion, before responding (or perhaps "owning up to" is a better choice of words to describe what he is doing) with a laconic, "I'm Episcopalian, I guess." He has for almost thirty years been married to a Jewish woman, whom he occasionally accompanies to a Reform synagogue, but only because he enjoys the services and admires the rabbi, with no hint of religious connotation to either of those likes.

Even Pete's canine preference is so different—and perhaps metaphorically so—from Miriam's as to deserve comment. Not only are they not loving little pets like Lucy, but the two aggressive Barker (and barking) dogs begin roaring at me the moment I appear in front of their house, throwing their powerful chests against the door as though determined to knock my intimidated body to the snow-covered ground and make lunch of it. They—both mixed-breed shepherds, one with a Doberman and the other with a Bernese mountain dog—have to be grabbed by their collars and locked in a bathroom before it is safe for me to cross the threshold, to the vast amusement of their apologetic master, who then smilingly turns his lanky form toward me and takes my limp and uncertain hand in a firm grip of greeting. Like their owner, the dogs epitomize vigor and reservoirs of energy, but, *un*like him, neither of them seems to have an ounce of affability or goodwill toward me. When my pulse comes down a bit closer to normal, I am ushered into a large living room pleasantly cluttered with the papers, books, photographs, and mementos of a life that has never slowed down enough to arrange itself into fastidious neatness. Though this is precisely the sort of atmosphere in which I am accustomed to working, I am mildly surprised by it, because I have been told that my host spent most of his career managing the finances of a large corporation. I soon learn that he has done a lot more than that.

The long peak of Pete Barker's career was spent as senior vice president and chief financial officer of CBS, a position for which he was well qualified by previous experience at a large petroleum company in Philadelphia and by his schooling at the Amos Tuck School of Business Administration at Dartmouth, where he had also taken his undergraduate degree. His first marriage took place in 1957 while he was a finance officer in the army (a job that did not prevent him from learning how to jump from airplanes with the paratroopers). Nine years and one son later, he and his wife divorced, soon remarried, and then divorced again in 1977, when Pete was forty-four years old. That same year, he married Gail Gottleib, who currently teaches broadcast and cable advertising at Fordham University's Graduate School of Business, following a successful career of her own as a sales executive.

Pete has been an avid track and field athlete all of his adult life, beginning as a senior in high school when he took up the shot put. He started doing judo at twenty-nine, and not only became a black belt nine years later but went on to compete in the Senior Nationals when he was forty-four. He transferred his affections to distance running at about that time. It was while training for the New York City Marathon in 1980, when he was forty-seven, that he noted the unexplained weight loss that proved to be the first evidence of the near-mortal disease that, twenty-five years later, would make him the subject of my interest.

Pete did enter the marathon, but had to drop out at the seventeenth mile because his back had begun to hurt so much that he found it impossible to continue. But back pain soon became the least of his problems, because he was also developing a fever that reached 105 degrees within the few days when he was trying to ignore his discomfort. Once his wife was able to force him to see a doctor, he was diagnosed with subacute bacterial endocarditis, an infection of the valve between the left atrium and ventricle of his heart. A long course of high-dose antibiotics cured the disease, but left him with a badly damaged valve that gradually became so incompetent that his heart enlarged, the ventricle weakened, and the heart's ability to eject blood dropped to 32 percent from a normal of more than 70 percent. After a time, even the most intensive medical treatment of the failing heart became ineffective, and open-heart surgery to insert a new valve was recommended. In 1993, the pathetically inept mitral valve was replaced by one of graphite. Except for an abnormality of cardiac rhythm called atrial fibrillation, Pete's heart has continued to function well, though it requires the help of a battery of pharmaceuticals. These include verapamil and two beta blockers, as well as a blood thinner to prevent clotting around the valve. In addition, a diuretic is needed in order to decrease the possibility of fluid overload that might lead to heart failure. Pete also takes Flomax, a drug meant to overcome an element of obstruction in a boggy prostate. Because of some mild pernicious anemia, folic acid and a monthly shot of vitamin B_{12} are also included in the regimen.

Another man might consider himself dependent on medications and hemmed in, or at least tethered, by the constant feeling of apprehension that the heart disease might slip out of control. But this is hardly Pete Barker's way. "I've had no morbid thoughts that my life has been shattered," he tells me, matter-of-factly. Pointing to his head, he adds, "It's up here. It's an attitude; it's what's inside your head. You could easily say, 'Oh my God, I'm a cripple.' But I've never done that."

From the outset, Pete's attitude toward having been so sick was fortified by the comments of his doctors, who not only refrained from discouraging his predilection for an active life, but supported it. "There was never any block put in front of me that said 'You shouldn't do this.' " So he did it, whatever "it" may have been at the moment of his enthusiasm. "Nothing seemed difficult to do; never was it suggested that I lie back, and no restrictions had been put on me." He has never thought of himself as a "patient," merely a vibrant man who periodically visits the doctor to keep everything in running order. He has never felt any need to integrate his experience of illness into a new philosophy of life. Unlike Miriam Gabler, a brush with death has not left him with revealed wisdom that he might not otherwise have attained.

Miriam and Pete share only one perspective about having come through illness of such nature and magnitude that it leaves powerful residues and significant potential for recurrence, a fact of which they are both very much aware: Neither of them thinks about being someone who might become sick at any time; they make no compromise with that knowledge. One has viewed her disease as an opportunity to grow, and the other as if it never happened, but despite such diametric differences, they share an equanimity free of morbid preoccupation.

Though Pete's illness has, like Miriam's, left permanent and indelible evidence of its depredations, his attitude toward them is to proceed as though they do not exist—in fact as though the illness itself was more a hurdle to be jumped than a near-catastrophe requiring course adjustment. All of this is manifest in the answer he gives me when I ask how his close call with death has influenced his attitudes about life, or changed him. "Quite frankly, it didn't." How different this is from the response given to the same question when it is asked of Miriam Gabler. "No, not at all," replies Pete almost flatly when I ask him if his joust with lethal heart disease has made life seem more precious. "I don't think a miracle has happened."

The proof of Pete's dispassion is indicated by the things he has done with his life since recovering from the first phase of his illness. Soon after the endocarditis, he took up running again, and it was not long after surgery before he returned, at age sixty, to the shot-putting he had done in high school and college. Since then, he has thrown the discus, the javelin, and the hammer, though putting the shot remains his favorite. He had retired from CBS in 1991, two years before the mitral valve replacement, and embarked on a series of business ventures involving television production, and he plunged back into them as soon as he had sufficiently recovered from the operation. None of these enterprises being particularly successful, he finally decided to think of himself as retired, in his late sixties.

In 1990, at the age of fifty-seven, Pete replied to a *New York Times* want ad for actors, and since then he has enjoyed a part-time semiprofessional career in film and amateur theater, including more than thirty plays and multiple appearances as a movie extra. With this added to his other interests, he is, in his own words, "much too busy." In addition to the fun and excitement of his acting career and all the time he spends training for the various masters' and senior athletic events in which he competes, he serves as lead director for two mutual funds and writes the newsletter for his Dartmouth class. And, of course, Pete being Pete, he finds plenty of other large and small matters requiring his attention, which keep coming up in the course of his bustlingly active life. As he punningly told me while describing his feats of athleticism: "That's what retirement can be: giving it a shot. You finally have the time and the freedom—you should try things you've never done before." He is a man on whom has been bestowed a super-abundance of things to enjoy. His life is vibrant, colorful, and quite obviously great fun.

And yet, it is the life of a man who knows that he is seventy-three, and takes account of it. But the accounting is less in terms of the number of years than in the messages he gets from his body, which his long experience of athletics has taught him to interpret so well. Relying on those and on his own good sense, he knows just how far he can go. "The things I'm doing," he points out, "are things I can continue to do. There are no artificial walls in terms of age." With care and prudence, there is no more reason he will have to give up any of the activities that bring him joy than there is reason that Miriam Gabler will have to give up hers. This is implicit in the answer he gives me—and only barely in jest—when I ask him what he looks forward to. He begins by describing the five-year categories of the Senior Olympics, which allow athletes to compete only with those in their own age group. Though smiling as he says it, Pete is quite serious when he describes his objective: "I'd love to set the world's record at the shot put when I'm a hundred." I reply with the obvious, "Let me know a few weeks in advance, and I'll try to arrange my schedule so I can come to cheer you on." Though I am two years older than the potential record holder, I am just as determined to be there as he is.

I already know the answer, but I ask Pete to tell me what

role faith has played in his ability to overcome illness. His reply is matter-of-fact, free of the emphatic certainty of some of those who are, underneath their air of assuredness, not quite certain. "Absolutely none," he says, and it launches us into a discussion of his real creed, which is humanism. Somewhere in the middle of it, I play the devil's advocate by posing the well-worn question of motivation when there is no God looking down with favor. Why does Pete Barker live a moral existence, why does he pay scrupulous attention to playing the game of life fairly and with regard for others, if there is no reward? Indeed, why should any of us? "Because it's the right thing to do," he says straightforwardly, as if the answer should be self-evident. He quotes a commencement address by Kurt Vonnegut that he keeps in one of the piles on his desk, in which the speaker tells his young audience that, as a humanist, he tries "to behave decently, without any expectation of rewards or punishments after I'm dead." Whether articulated by humanist or person of faith, it is a worthy credo, and one with implications well beyond selflessness. In fact, Vonnegut's—and Pete's—is in its own way a formula for aging. If there is a single factor that is the foundation stone for all successful aging, a factor that allows every other element, encourages every other element, and nurtures every other element, that factor must surely be a healthy self-image. We need to approve of ourselves, to take pride in what we have become, to feel a vibrancy in our moral sense—we must, quite simply, be happy with what we are.

None of this is to say that self-criticism and a bit of chronic dissatisfaction with ourselves as we currently are does not remain the bedrock by which the foundation must be supported. The fact is that none of us should ever be completely

"happy with what we are." If we are to think of aging as another stage in the maturing process of life, then it must also
be a stage of the continuing self-examination that may lead to
repairing the defects we find in ourselves and the world, or at
least those defects about which something can be done. Aspiring to something better is the restlessness we all need, a
form of energy that fuels correction of the factor that Miriam
Gabler calls "the part we play" in our own dissatisfactions,
and provokes the stimulus to the factor that Pete Barker calls
"giving it a shot." To be content, like Miriam, is not to be
inert, but to make the most of every opportunity within the
horizons she has drawn for herself. Nor is it to be so intoxi-
cated with one's own robustness—as some might erroneously
believe Pete Barker to be—as to become smug about all that
is being accomplished. Almost paradoxically, we feel better
about ourselves when we aspire to be just a bit better than we
are. What is meant by the "what we are" of the preceding
paragraph is thus seen to be "the kind of human being we
are," including openness to change. Like so many seemingly
hackneyed old aphorisms, "Every day in every way" is satu-
rated in truth, and holds unique significance for the later
decades of life.

Some aphorisms, however, hold up less well when scruti-
nized through the lens of reality, and those referring to good
deeds are particularly prone to prove windy. Despite the famous maxim, for example, the seventeenth-century physician-
philosopher Sir Thomas Browne was unquestionably correct
when, in his *Religio Medici,* he wrote, "That virtue is its own
reward is but a cold principle." Virtue without sensitivity to
the hopes and needs of others is a kind of self-satisfied steril-
ity, barely worthy of the name. Ironically, it is when we prac-

tice virtue in regard to its value to individual human beings other than ourselves that it rewards us the most. The reward is a happiness that sustains the self-image we need—at any age—for the peace of mind that nurtures the spirit. Here again, the words of Plato come to mind. In Book XLII of *Lives of Eminent Philosophers,* Diogenes quotes him as saying, "Virtue was sufficient of herself for happiness." Virtue, in the form of the good we do because of sensitivity to our fellows, can best be seen less as selflessness than it at first seems—less as selflessness than as the purest form of enlightened self-interest. It helps us to feel good about being "the kind of human being we are." Whatever else William James may have incorporated into the notion of pragmatism, this is a test of truth and values with which he would have agreed. We do, in fact, help ourselves by helping others. If there is a God who watches us closely, he surely knows that our reward in such things is as much on earth as it is in heaven—and sooner rather than later.

With all of this in mind, it would seem superfluous to ask Pete his thoughts about an afterlife, and it was. "I think you just stop" was his reply, and those words convey the lack of concern that he also shows for anything that will happen after death, including his heritage; he has never thought much about how he will be remembered. Like Miriam Gabler and everyone else I spoke to about such matters, he lives each day as a blessing unto itself—though he will doubtless phone me with vociferous objections when he reads this page and sees the word "blessing" associated with his name.

Pete shares with Miriam the sense that his response to illness, to life, to morality, to aging, is—and he uses the very word—"inherent." He believes that it arises of itself, without consciously needing to be called upon, from that vague mix of influences called nature and nurture that combine to form character. If this is so, it has no specific origin from one or several factors within that amorphous coagulum. Miriam might say the same about the basis for her inherent faith.

But in speaking to both of these thoughtful people, I find myself grappling with just that notion—the notion that one's response to life's circumstances is inherent, as though the word is synonymous with "immutable." I cannot agree with Pete when he tells me that his constructive reaction to adversity is necessarily the outcome of what he unchangeably is, any more than I agree with Miriam that hers has been guided by the hand of God. Human nature is far too complex for such simplistic explanations, and there are far too many shades of Eros and Thanatos in each of us—shades, respectively, of the life and death principles, of the optimistic and the morbid, of the need for guilt and self-punishment and the need for joy and the self-expression that leads to fulfilling happiness. As with the amorphous coagulum of influences that forms one's character, there is within us a disordered amalgam of impulses and instincts that are harmful and impulses and instincts that lead only to the good. It is not written in our stars or ourselves that we are compelled without option to respond to either good or bad in any fixed, predetermined, or "inherent" way. We have free will, whether we believe it to have been granted by God or granted by the very nature of the human mind. We are, in fact, capable of choosing how we respond to the circumstances of our lives, and in this way we are capable of changing them for the better— even when our initial impulse is counterproductive. Miriam says as much, though she attributes her wise choices to God.

I attribute them, on the other hand, to self-examination and the choices it has revealed to her. Though Pete has made choices too, his are less conscious, less deliberated. But he has made them nevertheless.

There are more than a few lessons to be learned from the lives of Miriam Gabler and Pete Barker. One of them is that choice remains, even in the face of adversity. To once again state the obvious: It is not the adversity itself that determines the shape of the future, so much as our response to the adversity. We have it within us to consciously and with deliberation choose a response that would seem to contradict what we conceive to be our inherent nature, if that course of thought and action is constructive and shows promise of leading to a better life. Especially when that course reverses an accustomed detrimental pattern of dealing with difficulties, the going may at first be rough, but sustenance can be found in the knowledge that the long-term dividends are great.

The difficulties lessen with each small triumph after the first few. Every hesitant trip to the gym, every tempting calorie reluctantly pushed away, every difficult refusal to allow rancor and self-righteousness their insistent demands, every small contribution to another's needs, every hour spent nurturing a relationship—all of these are building blocks to the gradually rising edifice of a changing, and in time changed, image of what we are. In the doing of these things we after a while begin to think of ourselves as the kind of people who do these things; we then do more of them. There is a pride in it. A sense of virtue in the context of such small beginnings thus does become its own reward, and we see our faces reflected in it.

Nothing encourages right living so much as the thoughtful, deliberate doing of it. Because we need successions of small successes in order to begin the process and keep it going, we must create them wherever we can, even if we have to drag our protesting selves kicking and screaming into action. Man is the only animal to have been granted the ability to continue developing during the later periods of life, and much of this depends on seeing oneself as the kind of person who can overcome the tendency to do otherwise. It is incumbent on us to use this ability.

And this is the real lesson of aging, or of any other stage of life. Whether it pertains to exercise, proper diet, creativity, goodwill, or the outlook and self-image that make all of them possible, choice exists for each of us, though it may sometimes involve a deliberate and difficult overcoming of lifelong tendencies or patterns in the opposite direction. Some of us are "inherently" more inclined toward making right choices than others, but no one except the most emotionally crippled of us are incapable of it. No matter the difficulty, it is necessary to reach into the complex of interacting and competing impulses and instincts, to choose those that promise later years of fulfillment and value to others. Once having made the decision to do what is necessary, the behavior must be implemented regardless of how difficult it seems at the outset. With time, it becomes an accustomed, glorious habit, as it is for both Miriam Gabler and Pete Barker.

FIVE

THREE WHO OVERCAME

I have written of prevailing over ill health and adversity—and, coincidentally, of making fundamental changes in ourselves—as though such victories must be achieved alone, the road toward attaining them traveled with only our own resources. Ultimately, of course, there is at least partial truth in that notion, because no one else can make the choice for us. Having made it, we must continue on that path, knowing that the determination to persevere does in fact come from some deep inner source that outside support may abet but cannot supplant.

That inner source may simply be dissatisfaction with what is. Or, paradoxically, it may be hopelessness that initiates a search for hope, because to do otherwise is to face a future of gnawing despair ending only at death. Sometimes, the source is a lingering pride, all but extinguished by the ruinous effects of an illness, or by despised traits in one's character. The strength for change and for overcoming hardship may even be found in that immodest extension beyond pride that we call vanity, which refuses to accept as unalterable reality the dissatisfied or even racked visage reflected from the mirror of each day's living. Or the source for change may be anger, which mounts into a productive rage of determination that the fates decreeing this assault on self-worth shall not triumph.

And sometimes, the inner source of perseverance consists of the conviction that we do, after all, live for others—it is for them that we need to seek something better. But the role played by others is often not as passive as merely motivating one's own pursuit of wholeness because a loved one's future will be diminished without our active contribution. The fact is that our own successful betterment is more often than not stimulated, encouraged, and made easier by those who hold our hands and steady our way as we take those tentative steps forward. On occasion, it is necessary that loved ones not do the holding gently, but instead so forcefully that they drive us into the only choice that can avoid their pushing and pulling, and their opprobrium if we hang back. They become drill sergeants in our lives; in order to accomplish their aims, they make demands, or even assert power over us. They know what is needed—and prod, rage, or domineer us into making choices we might otherwise not know we had, but for their hectoring.

Such a drill sergeant was the acclaimed writer Roald Dahl. The harshness of his demands may have grown out of his ac- customed ill-tempered irascibility rather than out of purity of motive, but it hardly mattered. The butt and beneficiary of his bullying was Patricia Neal, the Academy Award–winning

actress who was his wife; the occasion for his armed intervention was the crippling stroke Miss Neal suffered one
evening in February 1965, when she was thirty-nine years
old, pregnant with her fifth child, and at the peak of her career. Without Dahl's browbeating, she might have given in to
the stroke's devastating after-effects.

Miss Neal told me about these things on a January morning forty years after they took place, when I visited her in
New York a few days following her return from her home-
town of Knoxville, Tennessee. She had traveled there to celebrate her eightieth birthday at the opening ceremonies for a
new movie theater at the Patricia Neal Rehabilitation Center,
which is part of the Fort Sanders Regional Medical Center. It
is a place important to her, not only on account of its name
and the contributions she has made to its mission, but also
because she is well aware that her visits inspire the men and
women being treated there—they know how hard she had to
struggle in order to overcome her disabilities. "I try to make
them feel it's well worth the work," she said to a reporter that
day. "You really have to work," she told me during my visit.
"It takes so much time and effort, but you simply must do it."
Patricia Neal is an exemplar of her own teachings.

Sitting on the opposite side of a small kitchen table from
her, I try to mask the clinical appraisal of my subject that I
had promised myself to make. The residual evidence of her
stroke is only with difficulty visible to me from that perspective. I can detect none of the right facial paralysis that once
disfigured that extraordinary face, nor do I see any weakness
of her arm. Only when she had earlier walked into the room
to greet me, and later as she accompanied me to the door on
my departure, was I reminded that she has for forty years

lived with the restrictions imposed by a partially paralyzed right leg.

We are together in a small alcove between the kitchen and living room of Miss Neal's apartment on the Upper East Side of Manhattan. Her back is to a spacious window looking out on a traffic of small boats busily plying their workaday courses up and down the East River. Though most of the vessels appear to be tugs, scows, and delivery boats, the effect of the scene—with the majestically serene and quite beautiful face of a movie star of my youth directed toward me against the river-bisected skyline of New York City, set before the bright, brittle coldness of a winter morning's sky—is, to my admiring eyes, nothing less than magnificent.

As though conceding that it is out of place here, the brief foray into clinical detachment soon disperses itself and surrenders to the kind of youthful awe with which I might have viewed this stunning portrait half a century ago. Even the prosaic nature of the drab boats chugging their diligent ways over the rippling highway of densely black water is transformed by the aura enveloping my field of vision. Miss Neal speaks, and I hear the same voice that enthralled me all those years ago, with the same soft, perfect dignity of diction—though a few too many cigarettes each day for far too many years have made it a trace huskier than I remember, but for that reason even more alluring.

I have brought with me a brand-new digital voice recorder, but I forget at first to turn it on because I am mesmerized by the magically retained smoothness of the skin I am trying hard not to gawk at, still somehow youthful despite time and the cigarettes that usually leave so much wrinkled evidence in their wake; by the directness of the gaze Miss Neal has fixed on me with those clear deep-blue eyes (I would soon learn, to my surprise, that she is blind in her right visual field); and by that presence—she has not lost an iota of that presence, and it is no wonder that I am now so deliciously immersed in it that I have no wish to escape its spell. During our entire time together, I permit myself the perception of having been allowed within the gracious circle of radiance cast by royalty of a sort—specifically of a sort no longer known.

Though she does it tongue in cheek, as though acknowledging how far she has traveled since those long-ago days, Miss Neal still refers to herself as a hillbilly, a country girl born in the remote town of Packard, Kentucky, and brought up in Tennessee. She is of a time, a place, and an atmosphere from which American dreams were once made, and every gesture conveys her awareness—and enjoyment—of it. There is an openness in this, and it makes me like her almost from the first moment. Her easy smile and her comfort with banter convey her enjoyment of our time together, which makes my awed sense of her all the more magical.

Such is the web spun by Patricia Neal at the age of eighty, and she seems to know it. She chats, she smiles in bemusement and amusement, she speaks unself-consciously of the great and famous as easily as the rest of us do of our coworkers—for many of them were indeed her coworkers. And she tells with charming frankness of her feelings, her experiences, and the close attachments she has made, from the great love of her life, Gary Cooper, to Richard Daniel, who helped her up from the sidewalk in front of his shop when she fell one day, invited her in for coffee, and became her hairdresser, a pal with whom she would meet of an afternoon to share a cup and a few thoughts.

And she tells also of those terrible months four decades ago, after the bursting of a congenital weakening in one of her cerebral arteries let loose a small torrent of blood into her brain, one evening as she was bathing her seven-year-old daughter, Tessa. Aware momentarily only of an intense pain at her left temple, she staggered into the bedroom to get Roald, before collapsing into unconsciousness.

"I lay in a coma like an immense vegetable," she would twenty-three years later write in her autobiography, *As I Am*. "No one detects any movement in a vegetable except, per-haps, the shrewd gardener who knows its roots are reaching deep into the earth. So, perhaps, was my unconscious body reaching into the wellhead of raw existence."

She awoke days later in the intensive care unit of the UCLA Medical Center, having undergone a seven-hour oper-ation on the night of her stroke, to evacuate the blood and clip the offending artery to prevent further hemorrhage. Dur-ing all the time of coma, Roald Dahl was at her bedside, talk-ing to his unresponsive wife, occasionally trying to arouse her by slapping her face as hard as he could, and squeezing her hand again and again, until one day she squeezed back. That bit of squeeze was his first signal that she might survive.

When she first became aware of her surroundings, the confused, disoriented patient was completely paralyzed on her right side, unable to speak, and seeing double. But worst of all, "My mind just didn't work." As her thoughts cleared over the next few weeks, she realized that her husband had completely taken over. He insisted on telling her the details of her surgery, controlled the flow of visitors so much that some of her closest friends were forbidden entrance, decided which cards and letters she should be shown, and essentially forced her to make physical and mental efforts that she believed to be far beyond her capability.

Roald Dahl was an imposing man, and could be a forbidding one too. He was six feet six inches tall and was said by his wife to have "looked down on the world with deft authority." Dahl was born in Wales of Norwegian parents, and was a World War II hero of the RAF. He was shot down in Libya, crash-landed behind enemy lines, and through a combination of daring, quick-wittedness, and luck, made his way back to safety despite having fractured his skull during the crash. He later became a renowned and award-winning author of unconventional short stories and macabre children's books in which adults are often the subject of merciless revenge in retribution for their own cruelties. The most famous of them are *The Witches* and *Charlie and the Chocolate Factory,* but there are many others, most of them replete with menacing characters, ingenious and often bizarre plots, and plenty of puns and neologisms to spice up the narrative. They are clearly the product of a uniquely imaginative mind consumed with the sinister aspects of human nature and the underlying antagonism between the world of dark childhood fantasy and the stifling world of adult repression in which it is forced to exist.

If an author's writings are the key to his unconscious mind and a prediction of his behavior when challenged, Patricia Neal might have done well to listen to several friends who strongly advised her against marrying Dahl, including Dashiell Hammett, who told her, "He's a horror. I can't understand why you're doing this."

She explained to herself that she was "doing this" less out of love than because she wanted a family. And she was still on the long rebound from her intense affair with the married Gary Cooper. She tried to ignore Dahl's caustic wit, his never-ending need for admiration, his frequent rows with her friends and others, and an arrogance that demanded dominance over every situation in which he found himself. "Roald could be like sand in an oyster shell. He seemed to feel he had the right to be awful and no one should dare counter him. Few did."

In short, Roald Dahl was not a nice man, and Patsy, as her friends called her because it was her birth name, knew it long before she decided to marry him. But he had a certain élan about him that charmed her during the early days of his pursuit. And he was persistent. "Deliberate is a good word for Roald Dahl. He knew exactly what he wanted and he quietly went about getting it. I did not yet realize, however, that he wanted me."

It was precisely the persistence, the deft authority, and the ability to get what he wanted that would save Patricia Neal's future after her stroke. And, ironically, it was Dahl's wide streak of ill-disguised sadism, his almost brutish insistence that he be obeyed, and his refusal to be proven wrong that saved Neal's future. His very awfulness preserved her.

Both in the metaphoric and real sense, Dahl stood over Patsy with a pitiless insistence that she push herself beyond what she thought to be her limits. He accepted neither hesitance nor backsliding. Nothing would do but that she obey his dictatorial will that she recover. He demanded it, organized it, and oversaw each step in its accomplishment. Dahl found skilled therapists and helping hands of various sorts, watched over their work, and constantly sought new challenges that he ordered his struggling and uncertain wife to take on.

"I couldn't have done it without him," she told me. "No, no, no—not possible. He was so strict with me—he pushed me and pushed me." In time, and long before she thought she was ready, Dahl pushed her into making a movie. He did it not by his usual frontal attack but rather by means of a flanking maneuver. On New Year's Day 1966, he told reporters that his wife had said she felt certain of being ready to work within twelve months. "I felt nothing of the sort and was dismayed that he continued to press me to go back to work. He even got the Oscar down off the shelf and placed it smack in the middle of the sitting room window." He told her that she would never be fully recovered unless she went back to acting. "He insisted that I do the first film."

Reluctantly, Miss Neal signed a contract to make *The Subject Was Roses,* with Martin Sheen and Jack Albertson. When the filming began, she was still seething in anger at Dahl. "I didn't want to do it," she told me, grimacing a bit with the memory. "But by the third day of shooting, I began to be interested. Soon, I was feeling so glad he'd made me act again." She was enjoying herself, and knew that she was on her way. "Roald the slave driver, Roald the bastard, with his relentless scourge, Roald the Rotten, as I had called him more than once, had thrown me back into deep water. Where I belonged."

Dahl had one ally in his unyielding campaign: his wife's anger at all that had befallen her. "I was the most angry woman in the world," she recalled, smiling just a bit now, perhaps because the thought of it contrasted so starkly with her present serenity. "I was the most bitter woman you'd ever want to see. I screamed and cried. And my anger helped me."

Of course there were moments, even in the early days after the stroke, when the anger was forgotten: when so many of her good friends rallied to her support; when they helped her remember not only her accomplished past but the necessity to concentrate on the expectation of having an accomplished future, though she could not at first believe what they were telling her; and then there was that lovely day when Lucy Neal Dahl was born by a normal and surprisingly easy vaginal delivery on the beautiful summer morning of August 4, 1965—169 days after the stroke.

I asked Miss Neal whether faith had helped her, even in the midst of her anger. Though I did not know it at the time, she had addressed that question in *As I Am:* "I can remember what was left of my shambled brain bitterly reminding me that God had done this to me. And I hated God for that. I was angry and I would be angry for a long time."

In later years, the anger at God would dissipate and finally disappear, to be replaced by its opposite. "When I had my stroke," she told me, "I woke up not believing in one thing. I didn't think God could help me. But now, as time has passed, I must believe." It is unclear how far Miss Neal's faith goes, at least with respect to structured religion. Though not a Catholic, she has several times sought spiritual refuge for long periods of time in the nunnery of Regina Laudis in Bethlehem, Connecticut, where the tranquility and the wise counsel of the abbess brought her the peace and reconciliation that enabled her to write *As I Am* in the late 1980s. That book, from which several of these quotes have been taken, is dedicated "To my beloved Lady Abbess of Regina Laudis on her golden jubilee, for insisting that I remember it all." What is sensed in the book and in Miss Neal's presence is an abiding need for sustenance of the spirit and a deep conviction of God's guidance, rather than a systematic framework of belief.

That unquestioning conviction has clearly had a profound effect on her thinking.

> At the abbey, I was deeply impressed that God was using my life far beyond any merit of my own making. The stroke had been a means of allowing me to reach so many who were suffering. He had not given me the stroke. He was giving me the strength and love to move with it. I learned that my damaged brain cannot reclaim what is dead. It has to create totally new pathways that will allow me to make choices I would never have made had I not suffered that stroke—choices that an infallible voice assures me will be blessed.

But the notion of her choices being blessed must be understood in an earthly way, I think, for Patricia Neal seems unconcerned with rewards that might await her in some other world to come. What is important here is the conviction that it is her *choices* that are blessed, not herself. Those choices are made in the interest of other people. The reward is the happiness that sustains her sense of herself and her peace of mind, and nurtures her spirit. Plato was right— virtue is, indeed, the purest form of self-interest, and in this way is its own reward.

The fact is that Miss Neal has not thought much about any notion of afterlife, and assures me that she doesn't care whether or not there is one. And yet, she prefers to believe that something continues beyond the end of life. "I don't know, but I think we go on somehow" is the way she puts it. "I don't mind dying one bit," she continues, "because I've lived my life—I really have lived it. I'm so happy now. I really am, you know. So much has happened."

Patsy Neal of Knoxville, Tennessee, certainly has lived her life, and so much has really happened. One hundred thirty pages of her 403-page autobiography deal with the years after the stroke, and the book ends at publication in 1988, which indicates how much more has been lived since then. And much more time may yet remain in which to use her choices as an example to those who have benefited from her ongoing activities. Those 130 pages describe one ascension after another, despite the residual handicaps with which the stroke has left the author. I count performances in twenty-five motion pictures during that period, at least eleven notable television appearances, and numerous other professional undertakings since she made *The Subject Was Roses*. After that triumph of will and recovery, there was no stopping the onward course of Miss Neal's professional career. When I asked how she would like to be remembered, the validity of her answer was proven by the events of her life. "For my guts," she replied softly but nevertheless emphatically. "I refuse to be beaten. I've had a lot of stuff happen to me, and I'm still here."

That Patricia Neal has been "still here" and a very productive, happy presence for forty years following the episode that nearly took her life is a testament to sheer determination—hers and her husband's. She and Roald Dahl were divorced in 1983—he died in 1990—and everything she accomplished after that is to her credit alone. Despite her certainty about his role, whether or not she could, in fact, have begun on the long road back without his browbeating will never be known, but the woman I sat speaking with in that New York apartment had clearly made a choice early in her period of recovery, whether it came from something within or was, as she insists, forced on her by Dahl. In the end, it was her own stubbornness, her own refusal to be beaten, that kept her going even when she thought the obstacles facing her were insurmountable. Her remuneration has been the long years of middle and now older age in which she can say, as she did to me that morning a few days after her eightieth birthday, "I'm so happy now. I really am."

So much of Patricia Neal's life has been lived in the public eye, and she has revealed so much more in her candid and detailed autobiography, that an observer cannot escape reflecting on the effect that her fame may have had on the extraordinary recovery she was able to make. The wire services reported her death on the morning after the stroke, but she was soon afterward in the midst of what must have seemed a miracle to more than a few of her admirers, distant and close. Awareness that her progress was being carefully monitored by tens or hundreds of millions of people the world over must have added to the incentive not only to recover but, in more recent years, to achieve such a useful and rewarding older age. In a way, this puts her accomplishment into the category of one aided by the expectations and needs of others. But it only adds to the credit due to her alone if some of the armament in her battle was the driving desire to show the world that it could be done, and that she was the woman who could do it.

The influence of a watching world will be granted to very few of those who must overcome disability in order to achieve a fruitful old age. Were I to gaze as far as I could toward the opposite direction, I could find no one on whom it had a lesser effect than another person crippled by a stroke whom I met in the course of preparing to write this book.

Hurey Coleman is a tall, powerfully built African American man who works as a machinery operator in an industrial plant near New Haven. Strikingly handsome at the age of sixty-four, he is in his own way as attractive and interesting a personality as Patricia Neal is in hers. But other than his friends, his wife, their four children, and their seven grandchildren, the world will little note nor long remember what he did here. The incentive for his overcoming the massive stroke he suffered at the age of forty-eight was quite simply that he needed to get back to work in order to provide for his large family, but it was incentive enough. The strength and encouragement of his wife, Donna, and the children helped him considerably, but—unlike Patricia Neal—he never doubted that he would overcome his affliction. To his mind, continuing debility was not something God would allow to happen.

Mr. Coleman had never been very attentive to his hypertension. Not only had his doctor somehow not been able to hit on the proper medication to control it, but the patient himself was inconsistent in taking what had been prescribed. Late one Friday afternoon in January 1990, tired from having worked overtime at the plant, he came home and decided to wash his car. He was standing on the porch just after finishing the job when he suddenly felt the onset of severe pain in the back of his head. At almost the same time, he began to feel weak and dizzy, as though he were about to black out. To avoid falling, he sat down heavily on a porch chair, and then found himself unable to get up when he wanted to. Luckily, his wife returned from shopping only a few minutes later. When she saw that he was confused, garbling his speech, and immobile, she immediately called 911. On arrival at the emergency room of the Yale-New Haven Hospital, Mr. Coleman was found to have suffered a stroke that paralyzed his left side and made him aphasic—unable to express himself by speech or to fully comprehend what was being said to him. He spent twenty days at Yale-New Haven and was then transferred to the Gaylord Hospital, an inpatient rehabilitation center in the nearby town of Wallingford. And in that place, he resolutely went to work on his recovery. When he came home, it was with the determination to get back to work. Within four months of the stroke, he had done just that.

Mr. Coleman is justifiably proud of what he was able to accomplish. When I met with him and his wife in their neat, tastefully furnished house in West Haven, it had been fifteen years since the day of the stroke, and those years had been surprisingly good. But he still remembers how astonished everyone was at his rapid recovery. "Everybody was surprised at how fast I was able to do it," he said, with a touch of well-justified self-satisfaction.

But "everybody" does not include his wife. Donna Coleman works in the medical records department of the Yale-New Haven Hospital, and she had the opportunity to spend a great deal of time with her husband, watching his progress day by day. She knew from the first forty-eight hours in the hospital that Hurey would survive, and it would not be much longer before she also knew that he would do everything it might take to resume his normal life as rapidly as possible.

And all of this in spite of the extensive nature of the damage that doctors told her had been done to his brain, in the face of which so many men and women give up in despair and reconcile themselves to a life of debility. The basis of her certainty was faith in God.

"I never thought he wouldn't be able to go back to work again. They told me he was going to be a vegetable, or that he'd never walk again. But I never believed that. They thought he wouldn't make it. They kept telling me something negative and I kept telling them something positive. Positive thinking is important, and our faith is strong."

With that remarkable confidence—that God would bring him through—Hurey Coleman never questioned his part of the bargain. It was to work, work, work—and to remain cheerful in the assurance that all would be well. He did what he could to help others try as hard as he did, but he was not as successful in that self-appointed mission as he'd wished.

"When I was at Gaylord, a lot of the people there had the attitude—well, they'd just get so upset. When the therapists came to start the PT early in the morning—sometimes as early as five o'clock—those angry people would be swearing about having to get up, and I'd try to encourage them. 'We need this help,' I'd say. 'They can come and get me anytime they want. I'm not going anyplace anyway. As far as I care, they could wake me at three A.M. for therapy.' They thought I was a lunatic, but that's how I felt. I saw so many people give up and not cooperate with the treatment. What gave me strength was faith in God. That was what really kept me."

God had some pretty important help, not only from Hurey himself but from Donna and their children. "By my having a good wife and my children always coming to see about me, the family got even closer than before. We got strength from each other."

Mr. Coleman has been left with a somewhat weakened left arm and leg, and he uses a cane to steady himself when he walks. But he still goes to work every day, doing the same kind of job he did before the stroke, and he is obviously pleased with the way his life has turned out. When he says, "Everything has been pretty good. Everything is fine," there is plenty of evidence to show that his assessment is accurate. Of course, his activities are restricted somewhat by the weakness, and he can no longer go fishing as he used to, except rarely and then from a boat. Life has slowed down. But he still spends plenty of time with his friends, both with the men and with Donna as a couple, enjoys his family even more than before, and is considering—but only considering—whether to retire next year.

"I'd like to do more traveling—taking vacations. We're looking into a cruise, and we've never done that before. I'm thinking about retiring next year when I'm sixty-five. That way, I won't have to hit no more clocks, and I can do what I want."

Hurey's attitude is reinforced by the way he sees himself. I have spoken to many men and women who have overcome major health problems and gone on to rewarding later years, and one characteristic unites them all: The crisis was an event in their past, now behind them and perhaps necessitating certain changes in their lives, but not something that marks them as sick people. For some, the overcoming of the episode has become a subsequent source of strength; for others, it has seemed in retrospect merely a bump in the road; for still others, it has been a wake-up call to care better for themselves, or even to radically alter their approach to the necessity of maintenance. But none of these successful people—not a single one—considers her- or himself in any way invalided.

Even a man like Hurey Coleman, who every day has to take a total of ten different medications to maintain the stability of his heart, blood pressure, and kidneys, and who makes regular and frequent visits to Dr. Leo Cooncy, the director of Yale's Dorothy Adler Geriatric Assessment Center, who has cared for him since his stroke—even such a man is not seen through his own eyes as less than well. And there is no time or energy wasted on bitterness. "I never thought of myself as someone who is sick. I think of myself as a healthy man who had this problem. I've never gotten angry about it, or about anything else that was big in my life."

When I ask Mr. Coleman how he would advise someone recently recovering from the acute effects of a stroke, his reply combines his own religious beliefs and the practical plan he himself follows. Both have stood him in good stead through the years.

"The first thing I would try to do is to tell him to get faith in Christ. And then, go ahead and live a good life. Thinking about what you might have done in the past, or what might have been—well, there are things you might have done different, maybe gone in a different direction. But once that [stroke] has happened, you just have to go on. Have faith in God and take whatever medications the doctor puts you on. A lot of people don't want to abide by rules, but you have to."

As Hurey said those words I could not help but think of a Frank Loesser song popular during World War II, said to have been based on an actual event that took place in the South Pacific. The song was called "Praise the Lord and Pass the Ammunition," for the advice being given by their chaplain to a team of sailors when their ship was being attacked by enemy aircraft. He urged them to pray, but he also urged them to shoot back vigorously, even joining them in their efforts. Keep the faith, Hurey Coleman urges, but keep the firepower too, for the Lord does indeed help those who help themselves.

Except for the notion of faith in a benevolent God, Hurey's words might well have been spoken by a man whose life, education, and socioeconomic status have been about as far removed from his as Hurey Coleman's place in the public pantheon is from Patricia Neal's. At eighty-one, Arthur Galston is the Eaton Professor Emeritus of Botany; an emeritus professor also in the School of Forestry and Environmental Studies; Senior Research Scientist in Molecular, Cellular and Developmental Biology; and a professor in the Institution for Social and Policy Studies, all at Yale University. At various times during his long career, he has done extensive research in Vietnam, China (where he was the first foreign scientist invited to work in the People's Republic), Japan, Australia, Israel, Sweden, England, and France. Though his scientific bibliography is lengthy, among the works of which he is justifiably most proud is a book he wrote in 1973, *Daily Life in People's China,* the outgrowth of a summer spent working in the Marco Polo Bridge People's Commune, located in the countryside about twenty miles from Beijing. He is a navy veteran of World War II, one of our nation's most effective spokesmen on the dangers of Agent Orange, and well known as a leading academic figure in campaigns against the sort of

injustices that are created when our federal government mis-
uses or overreaches its authority—the Vietnam War is an example. He taught Yale's first course in bioethics, which he
initiated in 1977, when virtually no such teaching existed in
science departments anywhere in the United States. His remarkable career has been spent in a whirling vortex of research, teaching, and activism.

But Art Galston's arteries are like anyone else's. He suffered
a debilitating stroke in 1981 when he was sixty-one years
old, and a cardiac arrest eleven years later. Recovery from the
stroke took six months of commitment to intense physical
therapy, and left him with a slight but noticeable limp and
some diminution of strength in his right arm, effectively ending a long-standing and passionate relationship with the
game of handball.

Recovery from the cardiac arrest involved high drama and
sheer luck. Driving to his laboratory one morning in 1992,
Art began to notice what he thought was indigestion, and decided to stop in at the nearby Yale infirmary to see if something could be done about it. After checking in at the desk, he
went into the men's room and was just stepping out the door
when he suddenly blacked out. As he was told later, several
nurses sprinted to his aid and found him to be unconscious,
pulseless, and in full cardiac arrest due to the sudden irregu-
larity of rhythm called ventricular fibrillation. Except perhaps for an emergency room, Art's heart could not have
picked a better place to stop. The defibrillator was rushed to
his side as he lay motionless there in the corridor, a few jolts
of current were sent surging through his chest to reestablish a
regular beat, and an ambulance was called. Intubated and his
survival still in doubt, he was sped to the Yale-New Haven

Hospital, where he was stabilized and later underwent a three-vessel coronary bypass operation.

I have worked closely with Art Galston for only about ten years, since our mutual interests first brought us together at the Yale Interdisciplinary Center for Bioethics, on whose executive committee we both serve. But his reputation around the university and in the greater worlds of science and public activism have for far longer been well known to me, though I was not aware of his stroke or of the cardiac disease until recently. In fact, I had always thought of him as one of the university's many vigorous and vastly productive emeritus professors whose rewarding later years were made possible by their good fortune in avoiding major illness or infirmity. A few months before I began working on this book, a colleague told me of the problems Art had had, by then including his wife Dale's recent admission to a long-term care facility because of progressive dementia.

When Art and I spoke about these things, he had been living for several months in an apartment at Whitney Center, a comfortable and very homelike retirement community in my own town of Hamden, about two miles from the center of the university. The house in which he and Dale had brought up their two children—Beth, a sculptor, and Bill, a professor of philosophy and public policy at the University of Maryland—had been sold. Surrounding himself with some of the carefully selected memories of a lifetime, Art was determined to go on as before. Given his long daily visits with Dale, work in his office, his writings and teaching, and his contributions to the activities of the bioethics center, he was so amply busy that I had to find time in his schedule for our talk.

Art was one of the first people to whom I spoke when I was

beginning to wonder about finding value in the later years, for men and women from whom serious illness has taken away so much. I had no idea that his thoughts would be echoed in the responses of virtually everyone with whom I would later meet. Not surprisingly, he was so articulate in presenting them that I have chosen to quote him extensively here.

When his stroke occurred, Art said, he was sure that his career was over, until he began thinking about all he would be losing if he let that happen. The words came easily as he recalled his ponderings during that time: "I loved what I did; I loved being an academic. I loved having a research project I was engaged in. Most aspects of the academic life were very, very appealing to me."

Looking back on the pleasure he had taken in his career helped Art to emerge from the depressed state of mind into which he had allowed himself to settle. Realizing that he wanted the pleasure and fun back again, he determined to exert at least some control over his future, and not just let things happen to him. The mere thought of taking such a step gave him the enthusiasm to start on some positive action, and before long his enthusiasm was on the march again. "My attitude turned on a dime when I realized that there was a way out."

But a good attitude would not be enough.

When I had the stroke, I was despondent at first, but when a way appeared for me to work toward something, when the will took over, it didn't just happen. I had to work at it. But success fed upon success as I applied myself, first with the therapy and then with my career. Capabilities were restored, and I was encouraged. Before long,

I was pretty much restored to the status quo ante. At sixty-one, I felt once again the young tyro on the make. I wanted to do things; I wanted to be active. I had remarkable support from my wife and children.

I was aware that this machinery we've been given runs down. And this caused me to make some real changes. I started to be more observant about my diet, and I no longer flogged my body. I substituted a morning walk for the handball, and I began to take rest periods late in the afternoon.

The thing I knew was that I couldn't stand a life of inactivity. The human spirit, whatever it is, had to have some aspiration that was bigger than me, something I had to work toward in order to achieve. So I knew I had to have an activity. I had had such a good time starting up the bioethics course in the biology department which was very successful. After I retired in 1990, that became even more important to me.

Art's career soon restored itself, though in a somewhat modified form. But following the heart attack in 1992, another reevaluation would be necessary.

After the cardiac arrest, I said to myself, "Okay, I've now had two major episodes and my mortality has become a little more real. I don't want to lead myself into activities I can well do without." In other words, I became a little more crafty in planning things I wanted to do. That required me to evaluate what it was that I really wanted out of life at the age of seventy-two and after these two major health problems.

I thought, "I'm still a vigorous, aspiring scientist-teacher-academic. These things have happened and they're little roadblocks on the way to what I want to do, but I've seen that I can overcome them and I'm going to continue to overcome them," and that's exactly how I still feel.

In one's eighties, the nature of overcoming may need to change with each passing year. Art Galston addresses this issue in a brief essay he recently wrote for a planned Yale book on aging: "Could I continue to operate professionally at the age of 85? If I could, what would career #3 turn out to be? . . . This issue still has not been resolved, but one conclusion seems clear: any formal retirement emphasizing inactivity is for me not a viable option. I find the world much too interesting to permit me to sit on the sidelines as a passive observer. So I continue to seek participation in some constructive activity that will keep my mind and body active as long as that is possible."

And so, in fact, what does lie in the future? When I asked Art what he looks forward to, his reply was of a piece with everything he had already said.

I know my powers will diminish—they *are* diminishing. I'm a little less steady on my feet; I have to use a cane. I appreciate being here at Whitney Center. I realize this is a place that's better for me than my house in Orange was.

What do I hope for? I hope to continue in the ability to have a life outside of Whitney Center. I don't covet a total existence determined by living here. I still have my car; I try to go to my office every day; I'm still an active teacher. I'm teaching an advanced course in bioethics for upperclassmen and I need to be sharp—you don't want to embarrass yourself before a group of bright Yalies. And I continue to do some writing. I've edited two books for the Institution for Social and Policy Studies based on invited essays. The third thing is that I wrote a botany textbook in 1960, whose fourth edition I'm working on with a collaborator who is now the senior author. Between the textbook writing and my own creative writing of the essay type, and teaching—well, I'm pretty busy and if possible I intend to stay that way.

Confronted with the profound religious faith of Hurey Coleman and Miriam Gabler, the spiritual sense of a benevolent supreme being expressed by Patricia Neal, and the utter rejection of such concepts by Pete Barker—and my own studied skepticism—I was more than a little interested in Art Galston's thoughts about God and the afterlife. I asked him what role religion has played in helping him regain his life after two such major threats to it. His answer was direct, and what I might have expected from a scientist—especially one whose research interests have been to explain the phenomena of growth and development in nature.

None. I have very little patience with organized religion. I must say, though, that having had close relationships with ethicists has brought me into contact with theologians for whom I have great respect, but that does not change my thinking about the existence of God.

I certainly don't think there's a God in heaven, sitting up there in the clouds. But I do ponder how it all began. I'm sure that there's a primal force of some sort. In the beginning, there was energy, that's all there was. And energy became matter. That's the way I look at things. The necessities propel us inexorably along the evolutionary path.

And being a biologist, I think of death as a part of life. I don't believe there's an afterlife. I think things just stop. I'm not afraid of death. Unless I'm suffering with some horrible, painful disease, I'll accept it. Of course, I can't guarantee that.

Even if "things just stop," a life's work lives well beyond the life itself. And so does the world's memory of us. How would Art Galston want to be remembered?

I'd like to be thought of as a dedicated and able teacher who advanced knowledge of his field, a man with the courage to espouse unpopular points of view.

I surprised myself by my willingness to stick my neck out. I'd like to be remembered as somebody with a little guts, who stood up for what he believed in and was willing to pay the price it sometimes cost me. Everything has its costs.

As I think back on Art Galston's saying those words, surrounded in his small apartment by the books most important to him and the mementos of a life dedicated to science and the rights of those whose spokesman he has often been, it is the word "costs" that forces itself forward into my reflections. What is its meaning in the pursuit of a rewarding old age? The fact is that we have a choice in whether or not to pay those costs, especially when they must be paid in advance. It costs us to prepare for aging when we are in our forties and fifties and would rather not think about it—so sure that our bodies are still running pretty well without much up-keep. It costs us when we are in our sixties and seventies and beyond and we must scrupulously carry out the maintenance that allows what we hope for. And it costs us most dearly of all when there is crippling sickness to contend with, and a long and demanding road back that must be traveled. But in fact, it costs only in the same way in which an investment costs. We may sacrifice time and energy and perhaps some other variety of capital during the period when the necessary work is being done, but value is constantly accruing and the ultimate returns come in the form of the invaluable gifts deriving from all we have done to earn them.

When the Preacher of Ecclesiastes enjoined his listeners to "cast thy bread upon the waters; and it will return ere many a day," he was departing from the generally grim and pessimistic tone of his philosophy in order to shine a small but very strong light on the necessity to think of the future, for it will come all too soon. "There is a time to plant," he admonishes us, and if we choose not to plant, we will never earn the dividends that brighten the "time to pluck up that which is planted." And that, ultimately, is the message to be read in the lives of Miriam Gabler, Pete Barker, Patricia Neal, Hurey Coleman, and Art Galston: Making the right choice pays off; the fortitude pays off, no matter its difficulty. The hard work is an investment; the overcoming is the triumph; and the years of contentment and contribution—the years of plucking up—are the reward not only for ourselves, but for everyone to whose lives our lives contribute.

SIX

A FRIENDSHIP
IN LETTERS

The companionable hike, the long lunch, and the rambling bull session are powerful inducements to thought, and they help produce staunch contributions to a book as it is being written. To write about aging requires not only the study and experiences of a lifetime, but of the lifetimes of other men and women as well, whether they are learned authorities or merely those accompanying us on the long journey from birth to the grave. When that other, shorter journey—the writing of a book—is interrupted to allow the author to rest and reflect, it must be done on the three-legged stool of facts, knowledge, and, one can only hope, accumulating wisdom. Each of the three is distinct from the other two; none of the three can be omitted without destabilizing the traveler in his ruminations.

Throughout the development of this book, one of the sources of all three ingredients of my reflection has been a colleague of some four decades, Dr. Leo Cooney, who founded and continues to direct the Section of Geriatrics at the Yale School of Medicine and its affiliated hospital, Yale-New Haven. He is not one of the companions with whom I have hiked or lunched, but I have relied on our bull sessions as a bulwark against error and as a fountainhead for the getting of wisdom. I have depended on his counsel since writing the section on aging in *How We Die* fifteen years ago, and he continues to add to my understanding of the issues with which I am grappling as these pages evolve. In the field of geriatrics especially, vast experience is needed if facts are to be transformed into knowledge, and knowledge into any degree of wisdom. I have learned nothing so well from Leo Cooney as I have the importance for aging men and women of the interconnection between their lives and the lives of others.

The supremacy of that concept over other factors in successful aging is epitomized in something Leo said while we were one day discussing those many studies demonstrating the importance of exercise in maintaining vigor of body and outlook. "But exercise is not the Holy Grail," he pointed out. "If there's a Holy Grail, it's relationships with other people. In fact, if you have to decide between going to the gym or being with your grandchildren, I'd choose the grandchildren."

This led into a discussion of the need for each older man and woman to maintain a significant role as a distinctive individual within his or her familial and social encirclement— to have purpose, to have value, to have dignity—not only in self-perception but in fact as well. Those who are younger owe this much to their elders; those who are older owe it to those who are younger that they live in such a way as to merit being valued. Always, it gets back to contributing to the lives of others. Always, there is a mutuality in it.

Had I ever any doubts about these notions—and I never have—they would have been dispelled by a series of letters in which I became engaged in 1994, about six months after the publication of *How We Die*. In that book, I wrote of the depression so often suffered by older people, and of the increased rate of suicide caused by it. According to a 2005 census report, approximately 20 percent of the aged are reported to be clinically depressed at any given time, and the actual figure is probably higher, because so many do not seek treatment. Ruminating on suicide is frequent among the elderly, and the actual act would no doubt be more common if means of achieving it were easier to access. It was about access and means that a woman wrote to me from an address in Madison, Wisconsin, in early July 1994. Her letter was handwritten in a neat, easy-to-read penmanship on sheets of lined yellow paper torn from a legal pad. After a few comments about the book, she closed her first paragraph with a sentence telling why she had written: "There is an important matter on which I seek your opinion. No, it would be guidance." And then she described herself.

I am Indian, a widow, seventy-three years old. I spend a few months every year in India, and the rest of the time in Singapore, with my only son, who lives there with his wife. I have two granddaughters. One is studying in the U.K., the other is doing research in biochemistry in Wisconsin. I am now in Wisconsin for a month. I return to Singapore on the 22nd of this month.

And then, the crux of the matter.

> It is about dying when one has lived a full life with both happy and sad experiences and feels that the capacity of enjoying life is slowly ebbing away due to old age, should not one end one's life? I think that would be a happy ending. My vision is badly impaired. I cannot see in one eye, in the other a very limited angle of vision. When I go out, I have to depend on somebody else most of the time. My hearing is failing also. The doctor said it was due to weakness of the auditory nerves. I cannot move at a fast pace. This is degeneration due to old age. I am going the path of your grandmother [whose acceleration into beginning senility and her death at ninety-six I had described in the book]. I fully realize how she felt. There is nothing wrong with my health otherwise. I feel it is time I should die. That is, I should end my life myself. I don't want anyone to know about it. It needs to be done secretly or it would cause pain to others. What is the easiest way to do it secretly by one's own hands?
>
> Oh, Dr. Nuland, I know it is foolish of me to write in this way and it is likely that you will ignore this letter. I will understand. But I also have a faint hope that you may show me a way out of the future that I would not like to face.
>
> Yours sincerely,
> Ruby Chatterjee

How should such a letter be answered? Which of Mrs. Chatterjee's inner forces could be called on to change her mind and mitigate her wish to die? Clearly, every sentence of my response would have to be wrought with care, in order to transmit not only my genuine concern for her but also the message that her life had value though her single-mindedness was preventing her from perceiving it. I wrote back hoping to find an untapped vein of hidden optimism buried within the despondency that might still be seeking a solution to her despair. I chose to think of her letter not as a cry for help in self-destruction, but as a cry for help to establish a connection with another person, who might understand and suggest a way out. I responded several days later.

Dear Mrs. Chatterjee,
Your very eloquent and moving letter has touched me in important ways. I hope that I can respond properly to it, and help you to understand the importance of your life as it is at the present time.

Sometimes, Mrs. Chatterjee, it is necessary that we live for others. Yes, it is true that the various incapacities that are taking hold of your body are due to the gradual changes of age. However, it is also perfectly obvious that you do not have any major disease process that is likely to cause you a great deal of suffering, at least not in the foreseeable future. As you describe your son and your granddaughters, and as I have seen Indian families who are friends of mine, I recognize the enormous importance that you, without doubt, fulfill in their lives. I cannot, with any conscience, suggest that as basically healthy a person as you, whose mind is clear enough to write such a beautiful letter, should even consider taking her own life.

You must live for the sake of those who love you, because they need you. They need not only the reassurance of your physical presence on this earth, but they need your wisdom as well, in ways that you may not really appreciate. I would have been devastated had my grandmother taken her own life in her mid-seventies, and it would have had a profound effect on my ability to face the future. What can I do to encourage you to think optimistically, with the assurance of how important you are to those few people who really matter in our lives, the few that surround us in the loving circle of a family and close friends?

Please think of the things I have said, and remember that your humanity and your life are a gift that you are giving. Also, please understand that I am telling you these things from a great deal of experience in such situations, as I have watched them develop over many years. You must believe me, and you must also believe in yourself.

Mrs. Chatterjee's response was dated five days later. It was only a single paragraph long, but its six sentences gave me some optimism that she had understood. The letter ended with words I had only hoped for: "How can I not believe you? I shall do as you say. Thank you very, very much."

I thought the exchange was over, and felt relieved that such a difficult problem had been resolved this way. But months or perhaps years of morbid thinking on debility and death are not dispersed with a single letter. Three weeks later, Mrs. Chatterjee wrote me from her son's home in Singapore.

If I were your patient in any kind of illness, my illness would just linger on because I would want you at my bedside explaining the truths of life.

You have said one should live for others. That is indeed the essence of happiness and peace. . . . But in real life there are some difficulties. Truly speaking, in my condition there is little that I could give to benefit any other person. When I was young, I could—and I enjoyed giving of myself. My husband was of poor health; shouldering the responsibility of running the household and bringing up my son was all mine. Although a bit of a struggle, it did not really weary me. My husband was bedridden for four years before he died five years ago. It was in India. It seems very far behind. All I do now is tend the garden and water the plants and occasionally cook some dish that does not always turn out a success. I read quite a lot and sometimes sew, which is for my own satisfaction. As time passes I will be a burden to myself and also to those who care for me. I wish I could spare them this distress. In the midst of these disheartening thoughts life still offers some joyful moments.

Your book and your letter reach deep into the mind and I cannot turn aside the message that one has to face the inevitable in the best way possible. I have been just rambling on, please forgive me.

I had to be sure that there would be no reconsidering, no backsliding into the disheartened torpor that sought relief in death. I replied with much the same message as in my earlier letter:

Dear Mrs. Chatterjee,
I was very pleased to receive your letter, and to note that you are now safely back in Singapore.

I will have to disagree with you that there is little that you can give to benefit any other person. Our very lives benefit others, simply by the security of their knowing that we are there. Think of this in your own experience—think of the people whose contribution to you was simply that they existed as stars in your firmament, because their presence in the world steadied you and gave you some sense of direction. I am sure that your granddaughters and your son feel this way about you. I am also sure that you make far more real contribution to their lives than you can imagine. Just try asking them someday.

Of course we are all (healthy, aged, and every category) a burden to others, but we are also a burden that carries with it sweetness and love. Such burdens are a joy, and we should therefore rejoice in falling into that lovely pattern.

You have said in your letter that if you were my patient in any kind of illness, your illness would linger on because you would want me at your side. Please think of me exactly that way. There are those who think of life as an illness. It's a very mild illness, in fact, but it does require a certain amount of doctoring, which we should accept from those we love and those who become our friends.

Please remember these things.

In response to this, I received a letter containing a new and worrisomely unrealistic element in Mrs. Chatterjee's argument: Why not seek death at a moment of ineffable happiness, so that such an instant would somehow be forever part of one's eternal existence?

She wrote:

I had this feeling once when in Nepal among the Himalayan mountains. From a particular point one could see the highest snow-clad peaks on a sunny day. Well, the fog had lifted and there were the mountains in their sublime beauty. The sight was breathtaking. I felt I had to capture this moment forever. I wanted to die at that moment so it would never escape me. You have not written of this aspect of death. At our happiest moments we wish to die so that happiness is forever. For those who die in such circumstances, should we judge them harshly? Provided, of course, that there are no duties left undone, no promises unfulfilled. I have to wonder if there is something wrong with my reasoning, my mind. Is it that mild illness in life which you have referred to in your letter?

Following on this, Mrs. Chatterjee returned to her earlier concerns.

In cases of taking one's life you have mentioned [in *How We Die*] cases where one is crippled or in pain when there is no relief. This is justified. But the knowledge that one is on the way to being crippled, is that not enough? What is the use of prolonging increasing pain and an accompanying sense of insecurity! Better to put a stop to it while one can do it without having to depend on anyone else.

Dr. Nuland, most of the questions that I bring up are probably very odd and do not concern most people. But I cannot help thinking of these. I don't know what else to say.

Of course, not only was this last concern of Mrs. Chatterjee's not odd, but it is, in fact, the stuff of anguish for so many people with progressive diseases of a neurological or other nature who foresee the inevitable debilitation and wish to ward it off by taking their own lives while they still can. It was important to respond to both of the issues that had been raised in this letter.

I apologize for not having written in response to your last, and very interesting, letter. The obligations associated with *How We Die* have once more quickly expanded and I have been traveling quite a bit, including a week out of the country.

Nevertheless, I think your fascinating question is answered without difficulty. We must never make decisions based upon an impulse of the moment, even when the impulse is based upon evidence of transcendent beauty. Decisions about irrevocable acts such as death are to be made after much concentration, thought, and philosophical cogitation, as we both know.

Also, I question whether any of us have "no duties left undone, no promises unfulfilled," the conditions that you make the proviso for death under happy circumstances.

Again, I will urge you to think carefully about what I have said, because I know you give a great deal of consideration to the problems we have discussed, and approach them with the kind of maturity we all seek for ourselves.

Sincerely your friend,
Sherwin Nuland

But my correspondent was not easily convinced. Though she was willing to agree with my objections to seeking death at moments of transcendence ("reading your comments on dying happy with no promises unfulfilled, etc., I felt quite foolish and rather ashamed of myself"), her next letter returned to a theme I thought had already been settled.

I was reading your previous letter in which you said yes we are all burdens to others but a burden that carries with it sweetness and love. But I have known cases where the family members really feel the weight of the burden and it is a relief when the old parent breathes his last. And people don't have very much time to sorrow for the departed. It is accepted in a very realistic way. Only when death comes early and unexpected is the grief intense and prolonged. I think it would be very sensible for aged people who have lived a full life to end their lives if they wished to, and feel it would not affect any person adversely to an appreciable extent. There will always be some sorrowing on the part of the loved ones, but that is expected and may be treated as a normal occurrence. I am sure there are many aged people who will gladly want to make their final exit. . . .

I feel very much that society should make some provision allowing the aged to end their lives if they so wish. There should be no stigma attached to it. My life is my own and I am free to do what I want with it as I would do with the material goods that I own.

Soon after, following five months of such correspondence, I was able to reply with a letter that I believed would finally

succeed in putting to rest the greater portion of Mrs. Chatterjee's determination to do away with herself. By then, she
was back at her own home in Calcutta.

I'm afraid that I can't agree with you when you say, "My
life is my own and I am free to do what I want with it as
I would do with the material goods that I own." You will
have to admit that comparing your life with your material goods is hardly much of an analogy. Life is precious, a
gift of extraordinary value which has been given to us and
which we in turn give to others, and not to be compared
to inanimate goods. I certainly don't believe that our lives
belong only to ourselves, and you know how I feel about
this particular matter. Once we have formed relationships, our lives become of great importance to others.
Their manner of mourning and external manifestations of
grief or lack of it often bear no relation to the deep
wound that they may be unconsciously submerging. The
mind has peculiar mechanisms to cover up injuries to its
integrity and strength. I believe a decision to die is a decision that cannot be made without its being shared with
those who do love us. It is also, in a sense, a community
decision as well. Unchallenged, many people might wish
to die, but after a reasonable communion with those who
care about us, those decisions are often seen to be griev-
ously selfish, and I don't think that's too strong a word.
    I do agree that on rare occasions (in my experience it
has been very, very rare) there is a reason to end one's
life, but that must be a reason that is defensible to those
whose lives are part of ours. I don't see anything about
your physical or emotional state that makes such a deci-

sion at all valid. As long as you can keep writing to me in that clear lovely handwriting of yours, with the depth of thought and emotion that you transmit, you are a woman who is very much a part of this world and makes contributions to it that are beyond your own ability to appreciate.

Please believe me.

The response to this letter came from Delhi, nearly a thousand miles northwest of Mrs. Chatterjee's home in Calcutta, where she had been for about a month, following her time with her son. She was planning to spend almost two months visiting her niece in that distant city before once more returning home. Though her letter did say that she had "been stupid and selfish in my attitude to life," it contained nothing else in response to what I had written. But she did report the surprising news that her son, Rames, was to be transferred to Connecticut from his job with Black & Decker in Singapore. "He expects me to spend the summer months at least in Connecticut. . . . Could I hope to meet you when I am in Connecticut?"

Any expectation that my letter had resulted in my having achieved the objective of turning Mrs. Chatterjee's thoughts toward the value of her continued life was dashed by a later communication I received on March 16, 1995. But there was now reason for cautious optimism. Though my correspondent chose to only obliquely address my arguments, her writing now began to take an unanticipated but, to me, a more hopeful turn. She continued to write about her worsening disabilities, but absent was any mention of the wish to take active measures that would soon end her life. And though continuing her formality of "Dear Dr. Nuland" in the salutation and "Yours sincerely, Ruby Chatterjee" in the conclusion, the body of her next letter spoke of the nickname I have had since early childhood, which she knew from reading *How We Die*.

Dear Dr. Nuland,

I am always writing to you pouring out my woes. Perhaps I should restrain myself in this matter. . . . I often think about you as Shep, not always Dr. Nuland. You are the only person to whom I can speak without any inhibitions. I know I keep harping on the same theme most of the time. But what else can I do? I can feel age increasing its hold on me slowly and relentlessly. My eyesight is getting weaker, my movements are extremely slow. Walking for more than fifteen minutes continuously is very painful. . . . I wish I could speed up this process so I can cross the threshold of one of the thousand doors in no time. [The epigraph to *How We Die* is a quotation from John Webster's *The Duchess of Malfi:* ". . . death hath ten thousand several doors / For men to take their exits."] There were some people whose death affected me in the sense that I lost a valuable friend. But that does not mean that I expected them to live to an age where life would mean nothing to them. The time comes for each of us. I would expect my family to accept the inevitable in a realistic way. I have decided that when I become seriously ill I will refuse all medical treatment. That would hasten the end. I know I am selfish. I don't want to die bedridden. But I also want to spare my family the pain of watching me sliding slowly down.

Another surprise awaited me in the next paragraph. This seventy-three-year-old woman, already much limited in her activities and facing what she thought was worsening so imminent that she had had to be convinced not to end her life only nine months earlier, had not only traveled alone from Singapore to Calcutta and then from Calcutta to Delhi and back, but was planning an extended trip abroad, to a place almost 6,000 miles from her home.

> I will be going to Nigeria in late April. It may be for three or four weeks. My friends there have been wanting me to visit them for a long time. They are a very nice couple— about the same age as my son and daughter-in-law. I know, of course, that in my physical condition I will miss most of the sights and sounds that make Africa a very special place. But what I can take in is enough to keep me happy.

But perhaps she would miss much less than she'd expected. In a letter of April 5, the day of her departure, she wrote:

> I am leaving for Africa today. My first stop will be at Delhi. Then it will be to Nairobi by Kenyan Airlines. It is possible that I will have an opportunity to see the wildlife there, as I will be in Nairobi for three or four days.

The opportunity came to fruition in the form of a safari in the national park. There is no indication of the form of transportation, but I assume it to have been motorized; even in my wildest hopefulness, I could not imagine Mrs. Chatterjee on an elephant. The tone of the letter conveyed the excitement being felt by Ruby, as my correspondent was now signing herself, no doubt because I had called myself Shep in the previous letter. So we had now progressed from Mrs. Chatterjee and Dr. Nuland to Ruby and Shep. I began to feel like a rescue worker talking down a potential suicide from the ledge of a high window.

> And there were elephants, lions, giraffe, zebra, and whatnot! The giraffe are really graceful animals, Nigeria has not much of game resources. It is more noted for its art and culture and music. The drums and stringed instruments are very interesting. There is a twenty-one-stringed instrument called the "kora." There are flutes also, made from millet stalks, bamboo, gourds, as well as animal tusk horns.

Reading these words, I could not help thinking about the memorable aphorism of the English novelist Charles Kingsley: "All we need to make us really happy is something to be enthusiastic about." Often, but unfortunately not always, all we need to drive away or at least to mitigate depressive thoughts is to know that a moment of happiness is on the horizon.

Another letter from Lagos three weeks later was filled with further interesting comments about Nigeria, its great game parks, its culture, and its people. Clearly, Ruby had done quite a bit of traveling within the country, and she made observations far keener than I might have expected from the dejected woman who had first written to me the previous summer. Though she had traveled to Lagos with a companion of her own age, she returned home by herself. The long and complex journey seemed not to have fazed her. In a letter from Calcutta dated June 7, she wrote:

I arrived here last week. It took me five days going through many airports, changing flights, to reach Calcutta. And I was on my own. The lady who was with me when going to Lagos stayed back there. Do you know, Shep, I can face the unknown now with much more courage than I could before.

She was to leave for Singapore in two weeks, stay there for a few days, and then proceed to Madison, for a visit with her granddaughter. Then on July 20 she would board another plane to the airport in Hartford, Connecticut, where her son would pick her up and take her to his home, "at a place called Woodbridge or something like that. They say it is near New Haven."

A stretch of the eastern border of Woodbridge forms part of the western border of the town where I live. Rames Chatterjee had bought a house exactly eleven miles from my home. Wonder of wonders—Ruby and I would soon meet.

It would not be entirely accurate to say that I had mixed emotions about the imminent arrival on my doorstep of a woman with whom I had formed such a close epistolary bond. The fact is that I desperately did not want to meet Ruby Chatterjee. To be in her actual presence would be to lose the geographical remoteness, the unlikelihood of direct contact, that until then had enabled the intimacy of our relationship, to which I might have hesitated to commit myself had I so much as suspected that we would ever find ourselves in the same room. To me, the impossibility of physical closeness was an essential ingredient of the emotional closeness we had achieved.

My wife, Sarah, felt no better about it than I did. Her main concern was intrusion. She was well aware that I had not learned that a surgeon's sense of obligation to make himself accessible to everyone who might need him is precisely the opposite of the necessary privacy a writer must guard if he is to get anything done. Answering every letter and lingering with strangers on the telephone is conducive neither to efficient working habits nor, and more important, to the freedom of time for a close family life. Sarah had come to accept the writing of many letters, but what was in her view the invasion of her home was intolerable. She urged me to tell Ruby that I could not meet with her.

For days, the two of us went round and round on this issue, our discussions made more difficult by the fact that Sarah had, appropriately, not read the correspondence and accordingly had no real notion of my concern that a rebuff might lead to a setback in Ruby's gradual coming to accept the reasoning in my letters. And there was the additional fact that my correspondent had written several times expressing her anticipation and excitement that we would soon meet. I received a series of her letters, first from Wisconsin and then from Woodbridge. I would respond each time with evasive vaguenesses, as in a note I sent to her in Madison: "I have been away a great deal of the time, in addition to having just moved into a new home. Things are rather up in the air just now, but perhaps they will eventually settle down. You will remember that we began our correspondence when you were in Madison, and that alone should be a cheering thought."

The evasiveness was not lost on her: "You write that Madison should have cheering thoughts for me as it was here that our correspondence started. Will it also be ending here? I suppose I should take a realistic view of the matter as all things, however good, come to an end at one time." Having said that, however, she then made it clear in the next paragraph that she would not be denied. "I hope things will settle down before long. Can we then get together?" It was now becoming a struggle between my determination to find a way out and her persistence.

Ruby's next letter had a Woodbridge postmark. She was now coming closer, literally and figuratively. Because I was still putting her off with claims, not entirely unjustified, of being very busy, she was now asking whether she could phone, and even suggested that I stop by if I happened to be visiting a friend whom I had unwisely told her lived on the same road as Rames. Both Rames and Ratna were busy with work and other obligations, so, Ruby said, "here I have nothing to do and I have enough time at my disposal." My guilt at disappointing her was gradually mounting, but a new, or rather a revisited, element was now creeping into her thoughts. "Connecticut is a lovely place. To give you my first impressions in coming here, I have to go back to the subject of death. Looking at the green wooded areas stretching out at the back of the house, I thought—this is the place to die, to lie under the cool shade of maples and oaks and rest in peace."

My unease with the thought of meeting Ruby was giving way to concern about the tenor of her thoughts, and I quickly scribbled a message across a sheet of office stationery and got it into the mail: "Call anytime. Sorry for the scrawl, but it's the only way I could answer quickly."

Ruby did not, in fact, call. Or if she did, I never knew of it. I guessed that she was hesitant to take that step, in view of what was not difficult to interpret as my ongoing reluctance to a meeting. But there was a poignancy in her next letter that overcame my foot-dragging and even Sarah's previously adamant refusal to extend an invitation.

> You are so close—only twenty minutes away, yet I cannot reach you, such is the irony of Fate. After crossing more than half of the world to come here and hoping to see you, here I am sitting helpless, not knowing when I will be able to see you. I came for a four-month stay and already nearly two months have passed so quickly. This feeling of helplessness stems from aging. I just have to accept it, and the maples and oaks are there for me to rest in their shade. No, I am not thinking of dying.

A four-month stay! I had thought I would need to wait Ruby out for only about six weeks, and had been successful in that strategy. Four months, though, was beyond my capacity to keep delaying. But of even more consequence to my decision was the thought of the pain I was causing this increasingly disheartened and emotionally frail elderly woman to whom I had become so attached. She had in so many ways become my friend, someone about whom I cared deeply. And yet here I was, behaving as though the only thing of concern to me was my own privacy, and the notion that our relationship required distance if it was to continue to be valued by both of us. In view of the entire emerging picture of the forlorn, dispirited Ruby vainly seeking consolation from her lonely despondency under a Woodbridge tree only eleven miles from me, and the forlorn, guilt-ridden me vainly seeking expiation for my growing guilt, my decisions up to this point were more and more appearing to have been ill-advised. I showed this last letter to Sarah, and she immediately agreed that the time had come to change her mind.

I called the Woodbridge phone number in Ruby's letter. Within a minute, Ratna and I had arranged for the three Chatterjees to visit my home the following evening. The long period of avoiding the moment had come to an end. After more than a year of intense correspondence that had joined us fast to each other over a distance of 14,000 miles, Ruby and I would finally be in the same room.

In her last letter before leaving for the United States, Ruby had described herself.

> You have not seen me yet. I will give you an idea of how I look. I am somewhat overweight and wear thick glasses, and I wear Indian dress.

The description was, of course, completely consistent with everything she had previously written about herself, and conformed exactly with the image I kept in my mind each time I wrote to her. But now, with the moment imminent when I would actually lay eyes on Ruby, I unexpectedly found myself wondering. Many years earlier when I was in my twenties, unmarried, and working at Guy's Hospital in London, an Indian colleague asked me to come to a party at the home of one of his friends, where I would be the only person not part of a group whose members had known one another since school days. It proved to be an evening of high excitement for me, filled with unanticipated pleasures of a sort I had never encountered before. Adorned in a variety of filmy and quite revealing saris, their dark eyes flashing with an inviting warmth that was irresistible to a lonely young surgical resident an ocean away from home, the alluring girls I met made me feel the most desirable man on the planet. Even in the absence of liquor made taboo by Hindu restriction, the very spiciness of the curry and other exotic foods magnified the aphrodisiac spiciness of the erotically charged atmosphere pervading that small Shepherd's Bush apartment. There was just enough room to dance, providing that the partners held each other closely so as to occupy the smallest space possible. I took a turn with several of the girls, choosing from among the more enticingly forward of a bevy that seemed to me on that glorious evening the most beautiful, the most sensual, group of women I had ever seen gathered in one place. Holding one or another of them snuggled in my arms, I imagined that they wore nothing under their silken saris. I felt like a priapic satyr in a field of willing maidens. It was one of the most deliciously intoxicating evenings I had ever spent in my life, made more so by the tickling frustration of the impossibility, at least at the moment, of some consummation for my runaway libido.

I had often thought of that evening, especially as the onset of late middle age made bygone youth seem even more halcyon than it perhaps was. But, as paradoxical as it may sound, nothing had ever brought it so forcefully to mind as the thought of meeting Ruby Chatterjee. I had always been puzzled by the dissimilarity between her description of her ailments and decrepitude on the one hand, and the youthful clarity of her handwriting on the other. I looked again and again at my collection of her letters, and wondered more each time I fixed my eyes on them. Another perplexity was the description of her various and sometimes complicated travels, which would have seemed to require a hardiness not to be expected in a seventy-four-year-old woman with so many physical problems, added to what I judged to be a chronic moderate depression.

All in all, now at the last minute, I began to be concerned that I might have let myself in for a scam. I had more than once heard tales of seductive and determined women inveigling their way into the presence and eventually the bed of an unsuspecting writer upon whom they had set their sights. The thought that this might be about to happen to me was worrisome, but perversely pleasing as well. As so many husbands do when wanting to purge themselves of an enticing fantasy, I told my wife of my unease. "What can I do," I asked in a voice I believed to be sufficiently plaintive and sincere that she would think I looked on the possibility with unmitigated horror, "if she turns out to be a beautiful young woman wearing a sari and no underwear? This could be a trick, you know." Sarah threw her head back and laughed loudly, with a sound and look that revealed not only her dismissal of such a possibility, but also that she was on to me. "You'd like to think so, wouldn't you?" she teased mercilessly. "Just forget about the whole thing. She'll be exactly what she says she is."

And of course, Sarah was right. Ruby stood there in the entranceway as I opened the door on the following evening, looking as though she had been blinded by the light. She was more than "somewhat" overweight, her glasses were thicker than just "thick," and she wore Indian dress, as did Ratna. She was, in fact, just as she had portrayed herself, but more so. Ruby was a short, plump Indian woman in Coke-bottle glasses and a sari. But more important, she was my friend Ruby, with whom I had shared so much.

Despite what might be inferred from the foregoing description of her appearance, there was a distinct elegance about this elderly woman who stood with such uncertainty in my doorway, as there was about her son and daughter-in-law. Rames and Ratna were a handsome and self-assured couple, as I had somehow known they would be. My wife and I welcomed them into the house with a warmth I had not anticipated during the weeks of shilly-shallying prior to this moment. Now at this climactic instant in our relationship, I was immensely pleased that Ruby and I were finally together.

The group of us stood on the threshold—literally and figuratively on the threshold—for only a few moments, until an initial awkwardness faded. I felt as though I were a guide to a maharani's retinue as I ushered the Chatterjees through the central hall of my house and out onto the screened sunporch overlooking Sarah's backyard garden. Ruby took a place beside me on the couch, turned her body in my direction, and began to stare wordlessly at me through lenses so thick that I could barely see her eyes. She hardly spoke for the two hours we were together. As the rest of us sipped our tea, munched on our little cakes, and kept up a lively chatter about matters great and small—mostly small—she sat transfixed as though in a spell, in awe less of me, I think, than of the moment. She appeared to be so overwhelmed by the actuality of having finally reached this time and place that the beautifully articulate gift of expression capable of composing the challenging thoughts in her letters had simply been shut down by the torrent of overpowering emotions arising from some deep place within her.

Or perhaps Ruby had so much to say and so many thoughts to bring forth that the very profusion of words was clogging the channel through which they were to flow; or perhaps the closeness and the moment were strangling an ability to communicate that could make itself known only from the safety of distance and an effortless spontaneity of thinking unimpeded by the actual presence of its intended recipient.

Ruby, still in Woodbridge, would later write to say that she had wanted to speak of so many things that evening, but "I preferred listening to what you were saying," which was the only sentence she has ever written, before or since, that I cannot bring myself to believe. Quite obviously, she had been mesmerized by the aura built up in her mind, and no amount of her rationalizing could hide it. Her first letter came only a few days after the visit, and expressed a truth I had not perceived until I read it on the small sheet of notepaper. Indeed, it was the essence of any relationship that has meaning to both who enter into it. "You have given me so much yet you have never thought that you were doing me a favor. And I have taken from you, but did not feel that I was indebted to you. It is as if the way of Nature."

Ruby and I had been talking to each other through the mails for more than a year. On the face of it, an outsider might think that my role was the dominant one, but that would be erroneous. True, I was in a kind of mentoring, or—to use the word with which she had begun our correspondence—a guiding, role. But every mentor and every counselor must surely know that such bonds form a two-way street, as meaningful at one end as at the other. Articulated in Ruby's letter was a truth I had intuited from the beginning, but needed to see written there in words so that I could fully appreciate its value: The relationships that sustain us are relationships of mutual giving; though the giving may at first glance seem to flow mostly in one direction, such an impression, if subjected to thought and scrutiny, is seen to be mistaken. When Leo Cooney talks about the critical importance of relationships with other people, implicit in his viewpoint is the notion of contributing as much as one receives, in whatever form it manifests.

If there is a single bestowal we need from others in order to maintain a sense of self-worth, it is surely the gift of understanding. We all want, we all need, to be understood. It is when others seem not to understand what we are that we question our worth to them, and in consequence our worth to ourselves. No one can live a solitary or a lonely old age when feeling understood by those who matter in his or her life.

The reason Ruby heard so well what I had to say in those initial letters was that she could already tell not only that I was taking her seriously but that she was being understood. One does not care to understand another person if one does not care for that other. That this is on some level clear to both parties was the subtext of Ruby's words in this most recent letter. The notion of doing favors, or being indebted, has no place in such a bond. Had I ever needed evidence that it was not my words per se but rather the relationship we were developing that was the instrumental factor in changing her mind about the value of her life, the proof was there in the three sentences of this letter.

And what had Ruby given me in return? "In return" is not the issue. There is no quid pro quo when considerations arise from a mutuality of regard. From her first letter, I had sensed in Ruby a kindredness, a concern with issues with which I had dealt in *How We Die,* specifically the concept of the value of life. She had become in our letters a partner in my ruminations, a medium of responsiveness to my thought. In these letters, I had found a friend who understood why I felt as I did. Here, there were no favors, and no indebtedness.

I am going on at length about this matter because it seems to me that much of the unhappiness associated with the older years is the unhappiness of not feeling understood. So much of the reward and vibrancy of the older years, on the other hand, is associated with being understood by other men and women about whose opinions we care. That was—and continues to be more than a decade later—the essence of what Ruby and I did for each other.

My two hours with Ruby Chatterjee on that sultry August evening in 1995 was the only meeting we ever had. But our correspondence continues.

And so does Ruby.

In the eleven years since we met in 1995, Ruby and I have exchanged many letters, and many thoughts as well. Rames and Ratna now live in Colorado, and Ruby has visited them in one or another of their American homes a total of eight times. During the course of several of these visits, she has traveled with them from Connecticut or Colorado to California, Utah, Chicago, North Carolina, Niagara Falls, and perhaps some other places she has not mentioned to me. In 2000, when she was seventy-nine, she traveled alone to visit her younger granddaughter in the United Kingdom, where she is studying medicine at Leicester. A year earlier, Ruby spent two weeks in Dubai ("It is a pity that the women are still behind the curtains"), again traveling alone. On six separate occasions she has made the thousand-mile journey to Delhi to visit her niece, most recently at the age of eighty-three.

During this time, Ruby's health has deteriorated somewhat with increasing age, but only slowly. Her eyesight and hearing are worsening, as is her arthritis. In the late 1960s, chronic arterial obstruction to her lower extremities began to cause calf pain when she walked, but this eventually cleared without needing an operation; she underwent gallbladder and bile duct surgery in 2003; and was treated for a rhythm disorder of the heart in 2004.

And through it all, Ruby's spirit has remained indomitable. I have never again gotten a letter in which she ruminates about death. On the contrary, some of her writings are nothing less than inspiring. When I wished her peace and contentment on the New Year of 1996, she replied, "Well, I do feel quite content and at peace." Soon after, she wrote, "The days pass as usual with happenings, some of which make me happy and some of which I have to ignore. I look forward to being with those whose company gives me infinite pleasure."

In the winter of 1997, Ruby was trying to decide which of two fascinating destinations she should choose, whether Dubai or Santiniketan, the site of a school founded by the Bengali poet Rabindranath Tagore. But leaving Calcutta proved to be impossible at that time, because she needed to oversee the extensive work required to refurbish a new apartment into which she was moving. When she told me of this, I wrote, "It does my heart good to read of your trying to decide whether to visit Dubai, Santiniketan, or some other nifty place. Coming from a woman who was planning to leap off the end of the earth only a few years ago, all of this is very happy-making for me. As you can see, there is a great deal to live for, and plenty of pleasure for yourself and others."

Some of our letters are newsy, some more thoughtful, and some are both. During these past eleven years we have exchanged details of travels, holidays, the births of grand-children, world affairs, and cabbages and kings. Just before Ruby's eighty-first birthday in 2002, she wrote to me,

> In my younger days, when I was thirty or thirty-five years old, I always thought that I would never live to cross sixty. But I have crossed sixty, seventy, even eighty. Death has perhaps forgotten me. However, in spite of minor problems, life still has its charms.

Twelve years ago, Ruby Chatterjee came face-to-face with the existential crisis whose various forms have afflicted so many, as the later years become the present years. Despite her expressed certainty that death was the correct path for her, the fact that she reached out to another human being is evidence that, somewhere deep in her heart, she was nevertheless seek-ing to be dissuaded, seeking some reassurance that life was still worth living. She was able to find that reassurance in the realization that she was someone of value to others, as almost all of us are. Except under rare circumstances, the sense of aloneness is mistaken. And even in those unique situations in which it is a reality, a reorientation of perspective can create new relationships and new bonds, and strengthen old ones. A fresh look may even bring fresh realizations related to Ruby's meaning when she, in understatement, writes, "Life still has its charms." These charms are to be found everywhere. Like the wildflowers we have never before noticed as we walk through a familiar field, they are ours if we are but willing to look at them. And they are ours for the picking, at any age.

Early in the writing of this book, I had a letter from Ruby, at that time eighty-four years old, telling me that she would not be traveling to the United States in 2005, because she was not feeling well, and her physician suspected that she was developing early Parkinson's disease. This setback was particularly disappointing to her because she had planned to visit Great Sand Dunes National Park in Colorado, with Rames and Ratna.

> Rames says it is a beautiful place. But too much traveling
> does not suit me anymore. I had been to Delhi in June for
> a month. I cannot do more than that. Here I keep myself
> busy with household work and go out for short walks.

These lines represented the first time that Ruby had ever given any indication that she might be slowing down. Reading them, I found myself reflecting on our long friendship, and then turning back to thoughts of its beginnings and its evolution, as the evolution was traceable not only in my memory but in her letters. As I read through them one by one, it seemed that the story they told was a kind of cautionary tale in reverse—a tale whose lesson is hope. Ruby overcame the despondency of pessimism and morbid introspection. In time, death forgot her because she forgot death. Thoughts of death were dispersed when she considered the richness that is life. In one of her letters, I found her translation of a quote from Tagore.

"When I gaze at the infinity that is you, and lose myself in its beauty and vastness, Death and pain have no meaning, they are insignificant.

"But when I turn away from you and centre on myself, Death looms large and pain overwhelms me."

Only once in all of our correspondence has Ruby ever written of faith or belief in God, which so motivated the philosophy of Tagore. In a letter of April 2006, she described the love and kindness that she has found in human relationships, and added, "That is why I have never needed to turn to religion. I find plenty of these humane qualities in people around me. This is known as godliness. I am happy." In the context of the letter in which the poet is quoted, it is clear that "you" refers not to a deity but to the divine power manifest in nature and in life: its vastness, its beauty, and its ongoing essence for all humankind. The meaning she has found in Tagore's verse is unmistakable, and it is her own.

After reading all of our letters in sequence, I wrote to Ruby, because that cautionary tale in reverse is a tale for everyone who has felt the sort of despair that made her lose sight of the significance of her life. I told her of this book, on whose writing I had embarked, and asked for her help.

I want to address a chapter of my book to people who find themselves overcome by despair as they reach their later years; people who are beset with such physical problems as you were, and perhaps with sadness and depression as well; people who believe that they can no longer be of usefulness to others; people who feel that the effort to go on is not worth making; in short, people who, like yourself, have reached a point where they would prefer not being alive.

As you can probably imagine, there are many such men and women in this world of ours, and I know they can profit from your experience, and by knowing of the worth you have found in the added years since 1994. Please help me do this, Ruby, because your message can bring peace of mind to far more people than you may imagine. These years of our friendship-from-afar have been important to me, and I know they can also be important to countless people whom neither of us will ever meet.

For the first time, Ruby's response arrived by e-mail, via Rames. She described the reasons "why I should go on living."

That my life was not for myself alone, but also for others around me, especially for those with whom I have a strong emotional relationship. [Our correspondence] made me understand that in spite of growing old and infirm, I still had the ability to give something to others. This sense of being able to give and not just take, makes living worthwhile. When the mind and brain still function, one can contribute even a tiny bit for the benefit of those with whom one has a relationship of love and trust.

On receiving this, I wrote to Rames asking him to put one additional question to his mother, so that she might again write out her response for him to transfer to e-mail. "Were an elderly man or woman in despair (as she was when our correspondence began in 1994) to approach her, how would she advise such a person? What are the sorts of things she would tell her or him, so that they might understand the value of life?"

Ruby's response came ten days later.

> If anyone in similar circumstances approached me twelve years ago, I would have advised them to do just what I was wanting to do. But [our correspondence] then changed everything. I came to know that things were not as dark as I thought they were. Now I would tell them that there is meaning in life. We should have patience and look at life from a different angle. I now try to avoid doing something that I would regret later in life. This regret can be very painful and it is better to suffer if [suffering] benefits those whom I love. This gives me more satisfaction than the little bit of pain that I have to endure. You know all of these things, Shep. This is nothing new that I am trying to say, [namely] that I should give more thought to those with whom I have a loving and emotional relationship. That is the essence of life. This is what keeps me going. I love to travel and visit interesting places but I can no longer do this. I enjoyed having good food but this is now severely restricted. What I have is more than eighty years of experience of life. What I have learned from this helps me face the future.

Reading these words, I found myself thinking of some lines from Robert Louis Stevenson's *Lay Morals:* "So long as we love we serve; so long as we are loved by others, I would almost say that we are indispensable; and no man is useless while he has a friend."

We serve, we are indispensable, we have value in another's eyes and therefore in our own. The sense of being needed is the sense of purpose we all must find if life is to keep its meaning. We must treasure one or more others, and in the treasuring be treasured.

What Ruby had acquired in her more than eighty years of life is that precious alloy of knowledge and experience that we call wisdom. She had learned nothing new from our correspondence, nothing of which she had not been aware for most of her life. But before we began writing, she had allowed her own good sense to become submerged in a flood of self-pity, and she had come perilously close to making a decision of incalculable inconsistency with the principles on which she had based her life, the principles forgotten in despondency. Her obsession with lost powers and acquired debilities had pushed her so deeply into despair's pit that she had not the will to make any attempt at rising above it. Those who have made upward gains out of the chronic muck of despond know how slowly they are achieved, proceeding as they must through the acquired habit of faulty judgment and the molasses of doubt. In this sense, they are rather like the attempt to change the counterproductive behavior of a lifetime, which is discussed in earlier chapters.

Ruby had our exchanges of letters to help her. For every person who can push him or herself upward unaided, there is at least one other who needs help, whether from a friend or loved one or from someone professionally trained. It was guidance that Ruby had asked for in her first letter, and there are circumstances in which that guidance requires someone trained to provide it. The role of a therapist in such a situation becomes the role of a friend. Sometimes the first evidence of ascent is the choice to seek help.

Whether from a best friend or a paid best friend, what must be achieved is the connectedness of which Leo Cooney spoke. If it has been lost, it will have to be found again. It is the food by which the spirit is sustained, the drink in which the cells of our soul must be bathed. We require relatedness to others, both as individuals and as groups. By this means, we avoid or overcome the dreadful aloneness, the sense of helplessness that the aloneness abets.

If we have allowed our lives and our relationships to attenuate and narrow to such an extent that our connectedness to others has frayed or separated, there is a reaching out that must be done, and repairs that must be made. When the ancient Hebrew sages inscribed their dictum of *tikkun olam,* repairing the world, they included the world within as much as the world without, encompassing the world of our closest relationships. The repair of severed relationships has no "use by" date. It is never too late to reach out and forgive others, and to forgive ourselves. What usually requires forgiving is not so much the presumed cause of the breach as having allowed it to magnify its significance beyond sense or reality.

As important as these matters are at any time in life, they assume massive proportions as we age. There is an inner stubbornness that must be overcome, and it should be recognized as the pernicious thing that it is. And there is a self-righteousness, too, which is as harmful to ourselves as to those who are its object. We like to think that we acquire sagacity with age, but every retained grudge is a clue to immaturity.

When I mull over the factors that contributed to Ruby's renewed sense of the reality of her life and that have continued to buoy her confidence that "life still has its charms," I am reminded of a brief speech recently given by a much-valued friend at a gathering to celebrate his ninetieth birthday. Michael Bessie is one of that small cadre of legendary New York book editors who thrived during what might be called the golden era of publishing in the decades after World War II. Were there a Hall of Fame for such things, he would certainly be in it. With good health, two titanium knees, and no possible reason to fully retire, he lives with his wife, Cornelia, in the small and very Yankee town of Lyme, Connecticut. The Bessies have long had the most elegant of pieds-à-terre, in a brownstone on Washington Square in New York City. Gathered in the apartment late on a blustery January afternoon in 2006 was a group of perhaps forty men and women—many within a few years of Michael's own age—whose presence represented milestones in his distinguished career and the close friendships it has engendered. At the height of the celebration the host delivered himself of a characteristically witty disquisition on any number of things, including not only the value of long friendship but also the secrets that one must know if he is to attain great old age and still feel that the world is his oyster. "It is important to now and then have an adventure," he said, "and by that I mean an experience where you don't know how it will come out." He had told me much the same several times in the past, so I knew that this was no mere toss-off, but rather a principle of whose validity he was certain.

Of course, such a notion hardly applies to everyone. In fact, the basis of Miriam Gabler's equanimity is the very opposite. She has found her contentment in peace of mind through ordinary things. She might well enjoy an adventure, but she hardly needs it as something on which to base her sense of purpose or her hopes for the future. And yet, it can do wonders for some to vivify an outlook and fulfill Charles Kingsley's dictum that "all we need to make us really happy is something to be enthusiastic about." Miriam is enthusiastic about the everyday things that smooth the course of her hours. She understands that what counts is less the what of what we do than the dignity and grace with which we do it. But many people need something explosive from time to time, and for them the advice of Michael Bessie is just right.

Ruby's adventures were the voyages she made unaccompanied. Whether their highlights took place on an African plain or within the complexities of airports in the course of traveling, she frequently had no idea how "it will come out." From her letters, I could tell how much she enjoyed the challenge inherent in the very unpredictability of her complex adventures, trying to make her way from one stopping point to another.

Michael Bessie spoke that day also of the need always to have a project. For him, a project is the undertaking of publishing a new book, but he does not restrict his meaning to projects at work. For approximately three years prior to his ninetieth birthday he was engaged in the entanglements of constructing a large library room adjoining his home in Lyme, to house the enormous collection of books accumulated over a long literary lifetime, until then stored in various places in both cities where he lives. A project is a kind of adventure, and vice versa. In addition to being her adventures, Ruby's travels are also her projects, from the day she begins to plan them through their execution and her return home. My first intimation that she was emerging from her existential torpor was hearing that she had been to Nigeria, an adventure if ever there was one.

Of the several lessons to be learned from Ruby's story, perhaps the one of most basic significance to those who are pessimistic in the face of advancing years can be expressed in a simple sentence: We must never allow ourselves the luxury of despair. There is a certain self-indulgence in giving up, and it takes great heart and strong will to go on when the clouds blacken, because the easy way is to give in to the pessimism. But as Ruby herself would agree, the fear of aging is usually worse than the aging itself. Before you conclude that your options are limited, you need evidence that you cannot do something, rather than just deciding that you cannot do it.

With so many proofs of that proposition, I hardly needed the one that came after that exchange of e-mails, but it pleases me immensely to have it: Ruby's next letter reported that she had recovered from what proved to be a temporary setback, and had been shown not to have Parkinson's disease. She was already planning her next adventure, traveling to London for three weeks to be with her granddaughter who is now living there, and then on to the United States, where she will have an extended visit with Rames and Ratna in Colorado. November 20, 2006, is the date of her eighty-fifth birthday.

SEVEN

ADDING CENTURIES
TO OUR YEARS

I have been dealing until now with life as we know it, in which aging is an inevitable accompaniment of being human, and the days of our years have a natural limit imposed by membership in the species *Homo sapiens*. Because individuals of that species are the only animals with awareness that they will one day die, the instinct of self-preservation and the fear of death stand always in the wings of their minds, like unwelcome intruders waiting to leap out onto the stage to disrupt the serenity of the ongoing performance of being.

Fear of aging is more than fear of decrepitude. Ultimately it is fear of death. Since the predilection to avoid death is inherent in every biological structure and system, from cells to fully formed organisms; since it is an underlying theme of natural selection; since uncountable trillions of trillions of physicochemical mechanisms have evolved to preserve the life of every plant and animal large or small; since everything in our structure, our physiology, and that extraordinary concept we call mind militates against giving in to death—as a consequence of all this, is it any wonder that humankind has always been obsessed with the notion of life extension and even eternal existence?

Some would go so far as to claim that religion developed among us in order to provide reassurance that death is not final, that something of us goes on. Belief in God is belief in the supernatural, and if there is a supernatural—especially a benevolent and caring one—there is hope for some form of living beyond the mortal shape of it that we know. In this scheme of things, destiny is circumvented by faith, and the instinct for self-preservation presents itself in the nurturing thought that our lives, in one or another manifestation, will continue. Seen this way, religion becomes the paradoxical product of an inherent biological drive. Neither we nor God need ever die.

The earliest records of civilization already provide evidence of a preoccupation with afterlife as a way of prolonging existence forever. But for some, spiritual or religious faith have not been enough—these people have taken action on their own. In every generation, our forebears have used the knowledge and technology available to them to conceive or devise methods meant to rejuvenate and prolong themselves. The primitive period, the Egyptian era, the classical age, the Middle Ages, the Renaissance, the scientific revolution, the Enlightenment, the birth of modern science in the nineteenth century, and the decades of revolutionary discoveries in the twentieth—all epochs of history have sought and found their own approaches through which to express humankind's need to deal with the inborn drive to deny death. Magic and incantations and then formulae and potions gave way after centuries to testicular extracts and surgical implantations of animal glands, all in the service of rejuvenation and its promise of eternal youth and therefore life. As science and its clinical applications became so remarkably sophisticated after the mid-twentieth century, the overt emphasis increasingly focused on rejuvenation from aging, but the unacknowledged basis for all strivings toward such enhancements remained the instinctual fear of senescence and death.

With the discovery of DNA's structure in 1953, the rules of the ages-old game underwent a radical transformation. It now became possible to think in terms of altering the genetic predisposition to aging. Sugarplums were soon dancing in the heads of more than a few of the less restrained of the molecular biologists, who began to dream of life extension to 250 years or more, by tinkering up the human genome.

On its most direct level, this effort might begin with a determined search to identify a gene that controls the aging process, and so modify its structure that the entire sequence of events would be slowed. In fact, a molecular biologist at the University of California, San Francisco, Cynthia Kenyon, has identified just such a "master" gene in the tiny roundworm *Caenorhabditis elegans*. That gene appears to regulate the behavior of many other genes, all of which are in one way or another related to the metabolic changes that result in senescence. By modifying this so-called *daf-2* gene, Dr. Kenyon has been able to extend the life span of *C. elegans* from its normal twenty days to more than six times that figure.

That there is no evidence for the existence of such a gene in higher animal species has not by a whit slowed efforts to find one, nor does it appear to have dampened Kenyon's enthusiasm for the academic and, one assumes, the financial bonanza that awaits her should one be discovered. She and others are partners in a commercial enterprise incorporated with a name that echoes evocatively down the corridors of time as Elixer Pharmaceuticals, whose goal is nothing less than to produce a pill to prevent or slow aging.

Equally tantalizing to some scientists—and investors as well—is the potential they see in a structure called the telomere, which sits almost like a cap at the end of each molecule of DNA. Each time a cell divides, the telomere decreases in length. This shrinkage can be stopped or even reversed by contact with the enzyme telomerase, which allows the cell to continue dividing and, accordingly, live longer. The application of telomerase technology has resulted in a significant increase in the number of times a cell in laboratory culture can reproduce before finally dying. Despite no shred of evidence that the shortening or lengthening of telomeres can in any way affect an entire organism or human longevity, teams of biogerontologists are avidly pursuing its possibilities as a panacea for aging, and the wallets of venture capitalists open widely to follow suit.

Neither the scramble to find a "master aging gene" nor the cellular efficacy of telomere lengthening has shown evidence of any potential to add so much as an hour to human life, but there is one avenue of research that has already proven its usefulness, at least as high up in the animal chain as mammals, and perhaps even in the mammal called *Homo sapiens*. I refer here to dietary restriction, which since 1935 has been known to extend life expectancy in rats. The rats under study were fed 50 percent of their normal caloric intake, but there is reason to believe that even lesser deprivation may have significant effects on longevity. The evidence for this comes from the study of Okinawans, whose average life expectancy of seventy-eight and eighty-six years for men and women respectively is higher than that of any industrialized society. This has been attributed to a number of factors, but none is considered more important than diet, especially because the island's residents take in a smaller number of calories and get less of their energy from fat than we do. In fact, their centenarians ingest 10 to 20 percent fewer calories than is present in the typical American diet. Substantial reduction in caloric intake not only adds significantly to length of life, but also slows aging changes in the musculoskeletal, nervous, and endocrine systems, and reduces the frequency of cancer as well as certain other degenerative diseases.

Though the biologic reasons for the success of dietary restriction are not yet known, several reasonable explanations, or a combination of them, have been invoked. It has long been well known, for example, that the body automatically slows its rate of metabolism when fed fewer calories, no doubt as a survival mechanism in the face of possible starvation. This slowing is thought to slow the production also of the free radicals that are the by-product of normal metabolism. Because they injure DNA molecules, free radicals contribute to the accumulation of the irreversible cellular damage that ages tissues and organs. Free radicals, incidentally, are the highly reactive oxygen-containing molecules whose effects are said to be combated by the antioxidant pills taken by so many hopeful people.

Another possible explanation, though more theoretical, for the efficacy of food restriction is that a diet low in calories may influence the expression of certain genes by switching them on or off, and that these genes in some way determine the rate of aging, à la Kenyon and her worms. Whatever the mechanism, it is by now well known that dietary restriction works, at least in a variety of animals from flies to mice. Though no long-term study has yet been done in humans, there is preliminary evidence from at least one small group of obese adults studied for a relatively short period of time that the technique results in decreases in insulin levels, body temperature, thyroid hormone, and damage to DNA, and decreases in all of these areas are thought to be markers of longevity.

Of course, the key word in such restriction is "severe"— or even "extreme" or "drastic." In laboratory animals, the amount of reduction is in the range of 50 percent, a figure that few men or women would tolerate for any significant period. At least for the present, such a regimen is a practical impossibility, but that situation could change. It may be that various drugs will be developed that by one or another mechanism make such a program tolerable for those willing to forgo the normative gustatory pleasures of life.

But whatever may happen in the far-off future, the one certainty with which no responsible scientist can disagree is that there is at present no medicine or pill of any value to combat aging, nor is there likely to be one soon, if ever. Even those optimistic researchers who, with dollar signs flashing in their eyes, have partnered themselves with investors and management teams to found companies with promising names that seem to ensure eternal youth and health cannot fairly claim that they are anywhere near their goals, whether in the laboratory or at the stock exchange. Some of our most experienced biogerontologists are convinced that no "aging gene" will ever be found. Others point out that manipulating telomeres has the frightening potential to unleash an uncontrolled torrent of cellular reproductive changes sufficient to vastly increase the frequency and severity of cancer at the same time that it leads us to as yet unpredictable influences on growth and development, not only in adults but in their offspring as well.

Though extreme caloric restriction would appear to have some real promise, it may very well be that the disadvantages associated with it will deter all but the most determined—or foolish—men and women from taking part in it. As for the present market in panaceas—ranging from growth hormone to injections of freeze-dried extracts derived from fetal cells— be assured that, the loud claims of irresponsible hucksters to the contrary, no modality now available has any usefulness, and some may be more than a little dangerous.

All of this has been heady stuff, but not heady enough for one remarkable man, whose vision reaches far beyond a mere few centuries of life. Aubrey de Grey thinks in terms of millennia, perhaps eternity. He believes that he has identified the molecular basis for aging; he believes that aging can be prevented with means that are at present barely—if at all— visible on the horizon but nevertheless not entirely impossible. De Grey would rearrange the responses of our bodies to the passage of time, to heredity, and to the biology of life, because he believes to the depths of his soul that none of us should have to die if we choose not to. At the very least, he

believes the process of aging must be not only stopped but reversed. It is by his description "repulsive," and the death that
is its outcome is "barbaric."

His choice of such vivid words reveals a great deal of what
must be understood about de Grey, and about others so obsessed with the inevitability of death that they become zealots
in their determination to thwart its designs. They would tran-
scend biology, ecological imperatives, and the very nature of
humanity all at once. To ponder the propositions of Aubrey
de Grey is to ruminate on the entire philosophy of that small
cadre of scientists who have convinced themselves that extreme life extension is a worthy endeavor—worthy of their
talent, worthy of the vast amount of money that would have
to be poured into it to the neglect of more immediate health
concerns all over the globe, and worthy of the traditional
aims of the scientific enterprise. In any study of aging, account must be taken of those who would seek to prolong our
lives far beyond its species-determined length, and perhaps
forever.

At the request of Jason Pontin, the editor of the MIT *Technology Review,* I traveled to Cambridge University in the fall
of 2004, to spend the better part of two days with de Grey.
The pages that follow are the story of my visit to England. I
have since then spent more hours in de Grey's company, at a
conference in Spoleto, Italy, in the summer of 2005, where we
spoke on opposing sides at a conference called "Altering
Human Destiny." Each time I hear him describe what to me
seems the science fiction of his worldview and his conviction
that life is a problem in engineering, I return to my own most
deeply held certainty about the biology of our planet: the ex-
quisitely delicate balance that allows it to exist—achieved

over the course of 4.6 billion years for Earth itself and 3.5 billion for the living things that swarm on it—and is never entirely safe from going awry. There are immutable laws in nature that have allowed life to thrive, and we violate them at our own peril.

It was Sir Francis Bacon, the father of the scientific method of reasoning in the seventeenth century, who wrote, "Nature, to be commanded, must be obeyed." But some fifty years earlier, Michel de Montaigne had already unknowingly fired off a preemptive response to the life-extending futurists who would appear in our much later era. He presciently cautioned his readers and posterity that men should not tamper with nature, because "she knows her business better than we do."

Wandering through the quadrangles and medieval bastions of learning at Cambridge University one overcast Sunday afternoon shortly after my arrival to visit de Grey, I found myself ruminating on the role played by this venerable place as a crucible for the scientific revolution that changed humankind's perceptions of itself and of the world in the seventeenth century. The notion of Cambridge as a source of grand transformative concepts was very much on my mind that day, because I had traveled to England to meet a contemporary Cantabrigian who aspires to a role in the history of science similar to those of Francis Bacon, Isaac Newton, and William Harvey. Aubrey David Nicholas Jasper de Grey is convinced that he has formulated the theoretical means by which our species might live thousands of years—indefinitely, in fact.

Perhaps "theoretical" is too small a word. De Grey has mapped out his proposed course in such detail that he believes it may very well be possible for his objective to be achieved within as short a period as perhaps thirty-five years from now, in time for many people now alive to avail themselves of its formulations—and, not incidentally, in time for his forty-one-year-old self as well. Like Bacon, de Grey has never stationed himself at a laboratory bench to attempt a single hands-on experiment, at least not in human biology. He is without qualifications for that, and makes no pretensions to being anything other than what he is, a computer scientist who has taught himself natural science. Aubrey de Grey is a man of ideas, and he has set himself toward the goal of transforming the very basis of what it means to be human.

For reasons that memory cannot retrieve, de Grey has been convinced since childhood that aging is, in his words, "something we need to fix." Having become interested in biology after marrying a geneticist in 1991, he began poring over texts, and taught himself until he had mastered the subject far beyond the field's mere essentials. The more he learned, the more he became convinced that the postponement of death was a problem that could very well have some real solutions, and given enough time, he might be just the person to find them. As he reviewed the possible reasons why so little progress in "fixing" aging had been made, in spite of the remarkable molecular and cellular discoveries of recent decades, he came to the conclusion that the nut might be far less difficult to crack than some thought. The lack of progress seemed to him related to a factor too often brushed under the table when the motivations of scientists are discussed, namely, the small likelihood of achieving promising results within the period required for academic advancement—careerism, in a

word. As he puts it, "High-risk fields are not the most conducive to getting promoted quickly."

De Grey began reading the relevant literature in late 1995
and after only a few months had learned so much that he was
able to explain previously unidentified influences affecting
mutations in mitochondria, which are the intracellular structures within which certain chemical processes release energy
for the cell's functioning. Having contacted an expert in this
area of research who told him that he had indeed made a new
discovery consistent with available data, de Grey published
his first biological research paper in 1997, in the peer-
reviewed journal *BioEssays* ("A Proposed Refinement of the
Mitochondrial Free Radical Theory of Aging," *BioEssays*
19(2):161–66, 1997). By July 2000, further assiduous application had brought him to what some have called his "Eureka
moment," the insight to which he refers as his realization that
"aging could be described as a reasonably small set of accumulating and eventually pathogenic molecular and cellular
changes in our bodies, each of which is potentially amenable
to repair." This concept became the theme of all theoretical in-
vestigation he would do after that time; it is the leitmotif of his
life. He became determined to approach longevity as what can
only be called a problem in engineering. If it were possible to
know all the components of the variety of processes that cause
animal tissues to age, he reasoned, it might also be possible to
design remedies for each of them.

All along the way, de Grey would be continually surprised
at the relative ease with which the necessary knowledge could
be mastered—or at least he himself found it so. And here a
caveat must be issued, a variant of those seen in television

commercials featuring some daredevil and seemingly impossible automotive stunt: "Do not attempt this on your own. It is extremely hazardous and requires special abilities." For if there is a single impression that can be taken away from spending even a modicum of time with Aubrey de Grey, it is the indubitable one that he is the possessor of special abilities.

As he surveyed the literature, de Grey reached the conclusion that there are seven distinct ingredients in the aging process, and that emerging understanding of molecular biology shows promise of one day providing appropriate technologies by which each of them might be manipulated. His certainty that there are only seven such factors—and that others are unlikely to be found—is based on the lack of discoveries of any new ones in some twenty years despite the flourishing state of research in the field that has come to be known as biogerontology, the science of aging. His certainty that he is the man to lead the crusade for endless life is based on his conception that the qualification needed to accomplish it is the mind-set he brings to the problem: the goal-driven orientation of an engineer rather than the curiosity-driven orientation of the basic scientists who have made and will continue to make the laboratory discoveries that he intends to employ. He sees himself as the applied scientist who will bring the benisons of molecular biology to practical use. In the analogous terminology often used by historians of medicine, he is the clinician who will bring the laboratory to the bedside.

And so, in order to achieve his goal of transforming our society, de Grey has transformed himself. His "day job," as he described it to me, is relatively modest; at the time we met, he was working as the computer support for a genetics research team, and his entire official working space was a corner of its small lab. And yet, he has achieved international renown and more than a little notoriety in the field of aging, not only for the boldness of his theories, but also because of the forcefulness of his proselytizing for them. His stature has become such that he is a factor to be dealt with in any serious discussion of the topic, to which he has documented his contributions through scores of articles in the scientific literature. De Grey has published in an impressive array of peer-reviewed journals, including those of the quality of *Science, Biogerontology, Trends in Biotechnology, Annals of the New York Academy of Sciences,* and the aforementioned *BioEssays,* among others.

De Grey has been indefatigable as a missionary in his own cause, joining the appropriate professional societies and evangelizing in every medium available to him, including one of his own making, the sponsoring of an international symposium. Though he and his ideas may be sui generis, he is hardly an isolated monkish figure content to harangue the heavens and desert winds with his lonely philosophy. In addition to everything else, he seems to have a remarkable talent for organization and even for his own unique brand of fellowship. The sheer output of his pen and tongue is staggering, and every line of that bumper crop, whether intended for the most scientifically sophisticated or for the general biology-interested reader, is delivered in the same linear, lucid, point-by-point style that characterizes his writings on life prolongation. Like a skilled debater, he replies to arguments before they arise and hammers at his opposition with a forceful rhetoric that has just enough dismissiveness—and sometimes even castigation— to betray his impatience with stragglers in the march toward extreme longevity.

De Grey's is a familiar figure at meetings of certain kinds of scientific societies, where he has earned the respect of many gerontologists and that new variety of theoreticians to which the press has given the name "futurists." Not only has his work put him at the forefront of a field that might best be called theoretical biogerontology, but he swims close enough to the mainstream that some of its foremost champions and researchers have willingly agreed to have their names on his papers, despite not being in agreement with the full range of his thinking. Among the most prominent are such highly regarded figures as Bruce Ames of the University of California, the University of Chicago's Leonid Gavrilov, and S. Jay Olshansky from the University of Illinois at Chicago. Their attitude toward him is perhaps best expressed by Olshansky, who is a senior research scientist in epidemiology and biostatistics: "I'm a big fan of Aubrey; I love debating him. We need him. He challenges us and makes us expand our way of thinking. I disagree with his conclusions, but in science that's okay. That's what advances the field." De Grey has by his vigorous efforts brought together a kind of cohort of responsible scientists who see just enough theoretical value in his work to justify not only their engagement but also their cautious encouragment. As Gregory Stock, a futurist of biologic technology currently at Princeton, has pointed out to me, de Grey's proposals create scientific and public interest in every aspect of the biology of aging. Stock, too, has lent his name to several of de Grey's papers.

De Grey enjoys popular fame as well. He is often called upon when journalists need a quote on anti-aging science, and he has been the subject of profiles in publications as varied as

Fortune, Popular Mechanics, and the London *Daily Mail,* and, more recently, the subject of television documentaries. His tireless efforts at thrusting himself and his theories into the vanguard of a notion that has been eternally fascinating to the human mind have put him among the most prominent proponents of anti-aging science in the world. And his timing is perfect. With the baby boomers—perhaps the most determinedly self-improving (and self-absorbed) generation in history—now approaching or having reached their early sixties, there is a plenitude of eager seekers after such death-defying panaceas as he promises. De Grey has become almost more than a man; he is an entire movement. And that movement epitomizes the ancient and perennial yearning for eternal life.

I should declare here that I have no desire to live beyond the life span that nature has granted to our species. For reasons that are pragmatic, scientific, demographic, economic, political, social, emotional, and secularly spiritual, I am committed to the notion that both individual fulfillment and the ecological balance of life on this planet are best served by dying when our inherent biology decrees that we do. I am equally committed to having that age be, as close as modern biomedicine will allow, our biologically probable maximum of approximately 120 years, and I'm also committed to efforts at decreasing and compressing the years of morbidity and disabilities now attendant on extreme old age. But I cannot imagine that the consequences of doing a single thing beyond this will be anything but baleful, not only for each of us as an individual, but for every other living creature in our world. Another action I cannot imagine is enrolling myself—as has de Grey—with Alcor, the cryogenics company that will, for a price, preserve a customer's head or more until that hoped-for day when it can be brought back to some form of life.

With this worldview, is it any wonder that I would be intrigued by an Aubrey de Grey? What would it be like to come face-to-face with such a man? Not to debate him—as a clinical surgeon I would be scientifically unqualified—but just to sound him out, to see how he behaves in an ordinary situation, to speak of my concerns and hear his responses—to take his measure. To me, his philosophies are outlandish. I would in time discover that, to him, mine are equally so.

With all of this in mind, I contacted de Grey via e-mail in the fall of 2004, and received a response that was both gracious and welcoming. Addressing me by first name, he had no hesitation in offering to give up the better part of two days to speak with me, and moreover suggested that we spend them close to the lubricating effects of invigorating fluids, as follows:

> I hope you like a good English beer, as that is one of the main (open) secrets of my boundless energy as well as a good part of my intellectual creativity (or so I like to think . . .). A good plan (by which I mean a plan that has been well tested over the years!) is to meet at 11:00 A.M. Monday 18th in the Eagle, the most famous pub in Cambridge for a variety of reasons which I can point out to you. From there we may (weather permitting) be able to go punting on the Cam, an activity with which I fell in love at first sight on arriving here in 1982 and which all visitors seem to find unforgettable. We will be able to talk for as long as you like, and if there is reason to meet again on the Tuesday, I can arrange that too.

The message would prove to be vintage de Grey, including its hint of immodesty. And in a similar vintage was his response when I expressed hesitation about punting, based on some friends' tale of falling into the Cam on a chilly autumn day: "Evidently, your friends did it without expert guidance." As I would learn, de Grey is a man who will not allow himself to be less than expert at anything to which he decides to devote those prodigious energies so enthusiastically trumpeted in the e-mail, nor will he allow himself to hide his expertness under a bushel.

Of course, to conceive of being the herald and instrument of such a transformation as his theories promise requires a supreme self-confidence, and de Grey is the most unabashedly self-confident of men. Soon after we met, this unexampled man to whom self-deprecation is not known told me without a breath of irony that "one must have a somewhat inflated opinion of oneself," if success is to crown such great endeavors. "I have that!" he added emphatically. By the time he and I said our goodbyes after our total of ten hours together over a period of two days, I was certain that there are those de Grey watchers who would with good reason question if the high regard in which he holds himself is at all inflated, rather than simply being realistic. Whether one chooses to believe that he is a brilliant and prophetic architect of futuristic biology or merely a misguided and quite nutty theorist, there can be no doubt about the astonishing magnitude of his intellect.

De Grey calls his program Strategies for Engineered Negligible Senescence, which allows him to say that it makes SENS to embark upon it. Here, in no particular order, follow his seven horsemen of death and the formulations for the breaking of each animal and its rider. An attempt has been made to present them in a form comprehensible to the general reader, but those seeking further and more detailed information might wish to consult his website (http://www.gen.cam.ac.uk/sens/index.html), where such is provided. The website also has references to the vast volume of literature he has produced.

1. *Loss and atrophy, or degeneration, of cells.* This element of aging is particularly important in tissues containing cells that have been thought unable to replace themselves as they die, such as heart and brain (see chapter 2, page 34). De Grey would treat it primarily by the introduction of growth factors to stimulate cell division and also by periodic transfusion of stem cells specifically engineered to replace the types that have been lost.

2. *Accumulation of cells that are not wanted.* These are (a) fat cells—which tend to proliferate and not only replace muscle but also lead to diabetes by diminishing the body's ability to respond to the pancreatic hormone, insulin, and (b) cells that have become senescent—which accumulate in the cartilage of our joints. Receptors on the surface of such cells are susceptible to immune bodies that de Grey believes scientists will in time learn to generate, or to other compounds that may make the unwanted cells destroy themselves without affecting others that do not have those distinctive receptors.

3. *Mutations in chromosomes.* The most damaging consequence of mutations is the development of cancer.

The immortality of cancer cells is related to the behavior of the telomere and the role of telomerase in maintaining its length. If we could eliminate the gene that makes telomerase, the cancer cell would die. De Grey's solution for this problem is to periodically (the suggested period is ten years, for certain theoretically based reasons) replace all the stem cells from which our tissues are repopulated, with ones that have been engineered not to have that gene.

4. *Mutations in mitochondria.* Mitochondria are the micromachines that produce energy for the cell's activities. They contain small amounts of DNA, which are particularly susceptible to mutations since they are not protected by being housed in the chromosomes of the nucleus. De Grey proposes copying the genes (of which there are thirteen) from the mitochondrial DNA and then putting those copies into the DNA of the nucleus, where they will be far safer from mutation-causing influences.

5. *The accumulation of "junk" within the cell.* The junk in question is a collection of complex material that results from the cell's breakdown of large molecules. Intracellular structures called lysosomes being the primary microchambers for such breakdown, the junk tends to collect in them and cause problems in the function of certain types of cells. Atherosclerosis, or hardening of the arteries, is the biggest manifestation of these complications. To solve this difficulty, de Grey proposes to provide the lysosomes of the involved cells with genes to produce the extra enzymes required to digest the un-

welcome material. The source of these genes is to be certain soil bacteria, an innovation based on the observation that animal flesh does not show accumulation of degraded junk when it is buried in the ground.

6. *The accumulation of "junk" outside the cell.* The liquid in which all cells are bathed—called extracellular fluid—may come to contain aggregates of protein material incapable of breaking down. The result is the formation of a substance called amyloid, which is the material found in the brains of people with Alzheimer's disease. To counter this, de Grey proposes vaccination with an as-yet-undeveloped substance that might stimulate the immune system to produce cells to engulf and eat the offending material.

7. *Cross-links in proteins outside the cell.* The extracellular fluid contains many flexible protein molecules that exist unchanged for long periods of time, whose function is to give certain tissues such qualities as elasticity, transparency, or high tensile strength. Over the period of a lifetime, occasional chemical reactions gradually affect these molecules in ways that change their physical and/or chemical qualities. Among these changes is the development of chemical bonds called cross-links between molecules that had previously been able to slide along one another quite easily. The result is a loss of elasticity or a thickening of the involved tissue. If the tissue is the wall of an artery, for example, the loss of distensibility may lead to high blood pressure. De Grey's solution to this problem is to attempt to identify chemicals or enzymes capable of breaking cross-links without injuring anything else.

Even condensed and simplified as they are in the foregoing paragraphs, it must be obvious that these are enormously complex biological problems and even more complex proposed solutions. At least some of the former may prove impossible to overcome, and all or a few of the latter may prove impossible to implement. Moreover, de Grey's descriptions are sprinkled with such vague notions as "growth factors" and "stimulating the immune system," which might very well prove to be little more than slogans in this context, as perhaps is the invoking of still-unknown "chemicals or enzymes capable of breaking cross-links without injuring anything else." In addition, it must be emphasized that not a single one of the seven problems has yet come close to being solved. In the case of several, such as the extracellular cross-links, promising results are being obtained by researchers—so much so that a company called Alteon, in Parsippany, New Jersey, has been engaged in clinical trials. In others, such as the prevention of telomere lengthening or the transfer of mitochondrial DNA to the nucleus, it is fair to say that molecular biologists can only speculate about the day, if ever, when these attempts will come to fruition. But de Grey is fazed by none of this incompleteness. It is his thesis that time is being lost, and nothing is accomplished by pessimism about possibilities. The "pie in the sky" that his formulations were called by one of the biogerontologists I later consulted is a tasty delicacy whose promise already nourishes de Grey's soul.

But the thought of possibilities was not the reason why I had traveled to Cambridge to meet Aubrey de Grey. It is for others to challenge his science and even the completeness of his understanding of the biological world to which he is such a latecomer. My purpose was something else entirely. In addition to taking his measure, my purpose was to see what sort of man it is who would devote the labors of an incandescently brilliant mind and a seemingly indefatigable constitution to such a project. Not only does the science seem more than a little speculative, but even more speculative is the assumption on which the entire undertaking is based, namely, that it is a good thing for the men and women now populating the earth to be provided the means to live indefinitely.

I arrived at the Eagle a few minutes early on the appointed day, which gave me time to record some of the words engraved on a memorial plaque near the entryway, reading "An inn has existed at this site since 1667, called 'Eagle and Child.' . . . During their research in the early 1950s, Watson and Crick used the Eagle as a place to relax and discuss their theories whilst refreshing themselves with ale."

Thus properly steeped in history and atmosphere, I entered the pub just in time to see de Grey through the window, parking his secondhand twenty-five-year-old bicycle across the narrow street. Narrow, in fact, is precisely the right adjective for the man himself, who at a bit under six feet one inch weighs 147 pounds, his spareness accentuated by a mountain-man chestnut beard extending down to midthorax that seems never to have seen a comb or brush. He was dressed like an unkempt graduate student, uncaring of tailoring considerations of any sort, wearing a hip-length black mackinaw-type coat that appeared to be borderline shabby. Adorning his head was a woolen hat of a half dozen striped transverse colors, which I would be told had been knitted by his wife fourteen years ago. As if to prove its age, the frazzled headgear (which was knitted with straplike extensions that tied under the chin) was not without a few holes. When it was removed, its owner's long straight hair revealed itself to be held in a pony-tail by a circular band of bright red wool. But in spite of the visual gestalt, de Grey cannot disguise the fact that he is a boy-ishly handsome man. As for the sound of him, being the prod-uct of a private grammar school followed by Harrow and then Cambridge, it hardly needs to be described. To an American, he is of rare fauna, and his distinctiveness was catch-your-eye apparent even there among his Cambridge colleagues.

Having seen a photo of de Grey on his website, I was pre-pared for my subject's appearance of spareness and even his laissez-faire attitude toward externals. But I was most defi-nitely not prepared for the pallor that accompanied them, nor for the intensity of those keen blue-gray eyes and the face in which they are so gleamingly set, the whole making for an ex-pression of concentrated zeal, or even evangelism, that never let up during our subsequent six hours of nonstop conversa-tion across the narrow pub table that separated us on that first day.

The website photo shows eyes so gently warm that I had commented on them in one of my e-mails. But I would see none of that during the total of ten hours we spent together, though it reappeared during the fifteen minutes during which we chatted with Adelaide de Grey in a courtyard between lab-oratory buildings after our Monday session at the Eagle.

Adelaide Carpenter de Grey is a highly accomplished American geneticist and an expert electron microscopist who is nineteen years older than her husband. They met early in 1990, midway through her Cambridge sabbatical from a fac-ulty position at the University of California, San Diego, and were married in April 1991. Neither of them has ever wanted to have children. "There are already lots of people who are very good at that," explained Aubrey when the subject came up. "It's either that or do a lot of stuff you wouldn't do if you had children, because you wouldn't have the time." At the age of eight or nine, and being raised as the only child of an artistic and somewhat eccentric single mother, he determined to do something with his life "that would make a difference," something that he and perhaps no one else was equipped to accomplish. Why fritter away resources in directions that others might pursue just as well or better? With that in mind no less now than as a child, de Grey has trimmed away from his days and thoughts any activity he deems superfluous or distracting from the goals he sets for himself. He and Adelaide are two highly focused—some would say driven—people of such apparent similarity of motivation and goals that their work, hers in genetics and his in life-extension, is the overwhelming catalytic force of their lives.

And yet, each member of this uncommon pair is touchingly tender with the other. Even our brief fifteen minutes was sufficient to observe the softness that comes into de Grey's otherwise determined visage when Adelaide is near, and her similar response. I suspect that his website photo was taken while he was either looking at her or thinking of her.

Adelaide, though at five feet two inches much shorter than her husband, looks his perfect sartorial partner, dressed in a similar way and apparently just as uncaring about her appearance or grooming. One can easily imagine them on one of their dates as described by Aubrey. They have walked from the small flat where they have been living since he took it over from his roommates when the two of them married almost fourteen years ago, and are now in the local laundromat talking science as the machines beat up on their well-worn clothes for yet another time. They are hardly bon vivants, nor would they want to be; they quite obviously like things just as they are. They appear to care not at all for the usual getting and spending—and even some of the normative emotional—rewards of living in our world, at a time when the name of Aubrey de Grey has become associated with changing that world in as-yet-unimaginable ways.

But six uninterrupted hours of compelling talk (most of it pouring out of him in floods of volubility, let loose by intermittent questions or comments from me) and the consumption of numerous pints of Abbot Ale still awaited us before I would meet Adelaide and be taken to the laboratory where de Grey performs the duties of his "day job." Very soon after we began speaking, an hour before noon on that first day, I asked him, rather preliminarily, why it is that the hackles of so many gerontologists and others who might be expected to be familiar with the science of his proposals are raised by the very mention of these formulations—even by the mention of his name, in fact. And right there at the very outset of our discussions, he replied with the dismissive impatience that would reappear whenever I brought up one or another of the many objections that either a specialist or the common man in the street might have to the notion of extending life for millennia. "Pretty much invariably," he curtly told me, their objections "are based on simple ignorance." Among the bands of dazzling light that de Grey will not confine to a bushel is his certainty that his is one of the few minds capable of comprehending the biology of his formulations, the scientific and societal logic upon which they are based, and the vastness of their potential benefits to our species.

The burden of much of my challenge to de Grey was that

he should justify his conviction that living for thousands of years is a good thing. For certainly, if one can accept such a viewpoint as his, everything else follows from it: the push to do the research beyond just elucidating the biological process of aging; the gigantic investment of research talent and money to accomplish and apply it; the transformation of a culture based on the expectation of a finite and relatively short lifetime to one without limits to its horizons; the perception—because rejuvenation inevitably occurs as a result of de Grey's proposals—that all human beings are physiologically much the same age; the changed status of all relationships within the family, which is, after all, the primary group in which personality is formed—it goes on and on.

De Grey's response to such a challenge comes in the perfectly formed and articulated sentences of which all his writings consist. For he does have the gift of expressing himself both verbally and in print with such clarity, completeness, and consecutive sequence of explanation—even if without conciseness—that a listener finds himself entranced by the flow of seemingly logical statements that follow one after the other. As is true in his own directed life, de Grey never rambles in conversation. Everything he says is pertinent to his argument, and so well constructed that one becomes fascinated with the edifice being formed before one's eyes and ears. So much is this true that I could not but fix my full attention on him as he spoke. Though many possible distractions arose during the hours in which we confronted each other across that pub table as people came and went, ate and drank, talked and laughed, smoked and coughed, I never once found myself looking anywhere but directly at him, except when going to fetch food—a meal for me and only chips for him—

or another pint. It is only when reflecting upon the assumptions on which all of his thesis is based, that a listener discovers that he must insert the word "seemingly" before "logical" in the second sentence of this paragraph. Here follows an example of de Grey's thinking:

> The reason we have an imperative, we have a duty, to develop these therapies as soon as possible is to give future generations the choice. People are entitled, have a human right, to live as long as they can; people have a duty to give people the opportunity to live as long as they want to. I think it's just a straightforward extension of the duty-of-care concept. People are entitled to expect to be treated as they would treat themselves.
>
> It follows directly and irrevocably as an extension of the golden rule. If we hesitate and vacillate in developing life-extension therapy, there will be some cohort whom we will deny the option to live much longer than we do. We have a duty not to deny people that option.

When I raised the question of ethical or moral objections to the extreme extension of life, the reply was similarly seemingly logical and to the point:

> If there were such objections, they would certainly count in this argument. What does count is that the right to live as long as you choose is the world's most fundamental right. And this is not something I'm ordaining. This seems to be something that all moral codes, religious or secular, seem to agree on: that the right to life is the most important right.

And then, to what would seem the obvious objection that such moral codes assume our current life span and not one lasting thousands of years:

> It's an incremental thing. It's not a question of how long life should be, but whether the end of life should be hastened by action or inaction.

And there it is—the ultimate leap of ingenious argumentation that would do a sophist proud: By our inaction in not pursuing the possible opportunity of extending life for thousands of years, we are hastening death. A sin of omission thus becomes a sin of commission.

No word of the foregoing quotes has been edited or changed in any way. De Grey speaks in formed paragraphs and pages. Those accustomed to being interviewed are all too familiar with how garbled they often sound when quoted literally or heard on a tape, requiring adjustments of phrases and sometimes entire sentences in order to make themselves understood if publication is contemplated. Not so for de Grey, who speaks with the same precision as he writes. Admittedly, some may consider his responses to have the sound of a carefully prepared sermon or sales pitch because he has answered similar questions many times before, but all thought of such considerations disappears when one has spent a bit of time with him and realizes that he pours forth every statement in much the same way, whether it involves some problem he has faced a dozen times before or something as commonplace as ordinary conversation while showing me the genetics lab where he works. His every thought comes out perfectly shaped, to amaze a bemused observer.

De Grey does not fool himself about the vastness of the effort that will be required to attain his objective. Nor does he seem fazed by my reminder that his optimism might simply be based on the fact that, having never worked as a bench researcher in biology, he may not appreciate or even understand the nature of complex biological systems. Or his optimism may be based on his not fully taking into account the possible consequences of his tinkering with what he sees as individual components. Unlike the engineering approach that he considers his main conceptual contribution to solving the problems of aging, physiological events cannot be approached as distinct entities to be worked on as though none of them has any effect on the others. Each of de Grey's interventions will very likely result in unpredictable and incalculable responses in the biochemistry and physics of the cells he is treating, not to mention their extracellular milieu and the tissues and organs of which they are a part. In biology, everything is interdependent, and all things are affected by everything else. Though we study phenomena in isolation to avoid complicating factors, those factors come into play with a vengeance when in vitro becomes in vivo. The fearsome concerns are many: a little lengthening of the telomere here, a bit of genetic material from a soil bacterium there, a fistful of stem cells— the next thing you know, it all explodes in your face.

His reply to all this is similar to his reply to so much else, whether it be the threat of overpopulation, the changed relationships within families and whole societies when everyone is essentially the same age, or the need to find employment for vibrantly healthy people who are a thousand years old. We will deal with these problems as they come up, he says, and make the necessary adjustments, whether they are in the realm of potential cellular havoc or the tortuosities of socioeconomic necessity. He believes that each of them can be retouched and remedied as they become recognized.

And de Grey does have some interesting notions of human nature. On the one hand, he insists that it is basic to humankind to want to live forever regardless of consequences, while on the other it is not basic to want to have children. When I protested that the two most formative driving forces of all living things are to survive and to pass on their DNA, he quickly made good use of the one and denied the existence of the other. Bolstering his argument by the observation that many people choose—like Adelaide and himself—not to have children, he replied, not without a hint of petulance and some small bit of excited waving of his hands:

> Your precept is that we all have the fundamental impulse to reproduce. The incidence of voluntary childlessness is exploding. Therefore the imperative to reproduce is not actually so deep-seated as psychologists would have us believe. It may simply be that it was the thing to do—the more traditional thing. My point of view is that a large part of it may simply be indoctrination. . . . I'm not in favor of giving young girls dolls to play with, because it may perpetuate the urge to motherhood.

De Grey has commented in several forums on his conviction that, given the choice, the great majority of people would choose life extension over having children and the usual norms of family life. This being so, far fewer children would be born. He did not hesitate to say the same to me:

We will realize there is an overpopulation problem, and if we have the sense we'll decide to fix it [by not reproducing] sooner rather than later, because the sooner we fix it the more choice we'll have about how we live and where we live and how much space we will have and all that. Therefore, the question is, what will we do? Will we decide to live a long time and have fewer children, or will we decide to reject these rejuvenation therapies in order that we can have children? It seems pretty damn clear to me that we'll take the former option, but the point is that I don't know and I don't need to know.

Of course, de Grey's reason for not needing to know is that same familiar imperative he keeps returning to, the imperative that everyone is entitled to choice regardless of the possible consequences. What we need to know, he argues, can be found out after the fact, to be dealt with when it appears; without choice, we deprive humankind of its most basic liberty. It should not be surprising that a man as insistently individualistic—and as uncommon a sort—as he is would emphasize freedom of personal choice far more than he addresses the potentially toxic harvest that might result from cultivating that dangerous seed in isolation. As with every other of his formulations, this one—the concept of untrammeled freedom of choice for the individual—is taken out of the context of its biological and societal surroundings. Like everything else, it is treated in vitro rather than in vivo. All of the de Grey formulations are based on the great assumption that biology and culture work this way.

A major factor in de Grey's success in attracting a following is one that is less about his science than himself. As I discovered during our two sessions of Abbot-quaffing at the Eagle, it is impossible not to like him. Despite his unhesitant verbal trashing of those who disagree with him, there is a certain untouched sweetness in the man that, combined with that uncaring appearance and the sincerity of his commitment to the goals that animate his life, is so disarming that the entire picture is of the disingenuousness of genius, rather than of a remote and self-promoting false messiah. His likability was pointed out even by the detractors to whom I later spoke. It is a quality not to be expected in such an obviously odd and internally driven man.

In campaigns that occur across the length of several continents, de Grey's purpose is only secondarily to overcome resistance to his theories. His primary aim is to publicize himself and his formulations as widely as possible, not for the sake of personal glory but as a potential means of raising the considerable funding that will be necessary to carry out the research that needs to be done if his plans are to stand any chance of so much as partial success. He has laid out a schedule projecting the timeline on which he would like to see certain milestone events reached.

The first of these milestones is to control the aging of experimental mice sufficiently to triple their life expectancy. He believes adequate funding will make this doable "ten years from now; almost certainly not as soon as seven years, but very likely to be less than twenty years." Such an accomplishment, de Grey believes, will "kick-start a 'War on Aging' " and will be "the trigger for enormous social upheaval." In an article for the *Annals of the New York Academy of Sciences* in 2002 listing seven coauthors after his own name, de Grey wrote, "We contend that the impact on public opinion and (inevitably) public policy of unambiguous aging-reversal in mice would be so great that whatever work remained necessary at that time to achieve adequate somatic gene therapy would be hugely accelerated." Not only that, he asserts, but the public enthusiasm following upon such a feat will cause many people to begin making life choices based on the probability that they too can reach an equivalent number of years. Such life choices include several that even a skeptic like me would look on with pleasure: For example, when people know that they may live as long as four to five hundred years (with ongoing research during that time sure to add multiples of such a figure), they will take fewer chances of involving themselves in anything that might kill them, like wars, crime, bad driving habits, and other hazardous activities. Not only that, but when death of a disease such as influenza is considered premature at the age of two hundred, the urgency to solve the problems of infectious disease will massively increase government and drug company funding in that area.

In addition to accelerating demand for the appropriate research on human applications, the survival of a nine-year-old mouse born to live a third that long is projected to bring in new sources of funding. Because governments and drug companies tend to favor research that promises useful results in a relatively short time, de Grey is not counting on them as a source. He is relying on an infusion of private money to supply the approximately one hundred million dollars per year that he estimates it will take to successfully fight his "war." It is his contention that once mouse-success has been achieved, billionaires will come forward, intent on living as long as possible and having the personal means to support the studies that might make it happen.

Of course, such an optimistic visionary would hardly call attention to the likelihood that quite the opposite effect might result from the appearance of a photograph of his long-lived mouse on the front page of every newspaper in the world. Is it conceivable that such an event would be greeted with the unalloyed enthusiasm of a unanimous public universally eager to open an unlabeled can of worms and begin eating its contents with such voracious appetite as he predicts? I doubt it. More likely, one man's acclaim would be at least one other man's horror. Ethicists, economists, sociologists, members of the clergy, and many worried scientists can be counted on to join huge numbers of thoughtful citizens in a reaction the likes of which would make the present uproar over human cloning seem like a genteel tea party. But, of course, if we are to accept the line of reasoning that follows so logically from de Grey's first principle, that the desire to live forever trumps every other factor in human decision-making, then self-interest—or what some, including me, might call narcissism—will win out in the end. I have more confidence in human nature than to believe that.

De Grey projects that fifteen years beyond the mouse may be enough time in which to reach the goal of tripling human life expectancy, though he concedes that it may take as long as a century. What he does not concede, of course, is that it is more likely not to happen at all. He cannot seem to imagine— considering all the realistic pitfalls along the way—that the odds are heavily against him. And he also cannot seem to imagine that not only the odds but society itself may not come out in his favor. So convinced is he that the inborn urge to conquer death is sufficiently strong that it supersedes any other consideration—including the possibility of destroying our civilization, just the thing that is meant to be enhanced—that he will provide any listener or reader with a string of reasons (more like rationalizations) to explain away why it is that most mainstream gerontologists remain so conspicuously absent from the ranks of those cheering him on. Despite his publicized face and the increasingly loud fanfare that attends some of his pronouncements, he has safeguarded himself against the informed criticism that one might reasonably expect should give him cause to rethink some of his proposals. He has accomplished this self-protection by constructing a personal worldview in which he is made inviolate. He stubbornly refuses to budge a millimeter; he will not give ground to the possibility that any of the barriers to his success may prove to be insuperable.

Many decades ago, in my naïveté and ignorance, I used to think that the ultimate destruction of our planet would be by the neutral power of celestial catastrophe: collision with a gigantic meteor, the burning out of the sun—that sort of thing. In time, I came to believe that the end of days would be by the malevolence of a mad dictator who would unleash an arsenal of explosive or biological weaponry: nuclear bombs, engineered microorganisms—that sort of thing. But my notion of the nature of "that sort of thing" has recently been changing. If we are to be destroyed, I have now become convinced, it will not be a neutral or malevolent force that will do us in, but one that is benevolent in the extreme, one whose only motivation is to improve us and better our civilization.

If we are ever immolated or ever self-immolate, it will be by the efforts of well-meaning scientists who are convinced that they have our best interests at heart. We already know who they are. They are the DNA-tweakers who would enhance us by allowing each set of parents to choose the genetic makeup of their descendants unto every succeeding generation ad infinitum, heedless of the possibility that breeding out variety may alter factors necessary for the survival of our species and its relationship to every form of life on earth; they are the biogerontologists who study extreme caloric restriction in mice and promise us an expectancy extended by 20 percent of a peculiarly nourished existence; they are those other biogerontologists who emerge from their laboratories of molecular science every evening optimistic that they have come just a bit closer to their goal of having us live 250 years by engineering genes, adjusting telomerase, or some other such strategy, downplaying the unanticipated havoc at both the cellular and societal levels that might be wrought by their proposed manipulations.

And now, finally, it is the unique and strangely alluring figure of Aubrey de Grey, who, orating, writing, and striding tirelessly through our midst and the midst of some less-than-fully convinced sympathizers, proclaims like the disheveled herald of a new-begotten future that our most inalienable right is to have the choice of living as long as we wish. With the passion of a single-minded zealot crusading against time, he has issued the ultimate challenge, I believe, to our entire concept of the meaning of humanness. And paradoxically, his clarion call to action is the message of neither a madman nor a bad man, but of a brilliant, beneficent man of good will, who wants only for civilization to fulfill the highest hopes he has for its future. It is a good thing that his grand design will almost certainly not succeed. Were it otherwise, he would surely destroy us in attempting to preserve us.

EIGHT

DRINKING FROM THE
FOUNTAIN OF YOUTH

I sometimes find myself thinking about a long-dead French-man named Brown-Séquard, whose distinguished reputa-tion as a medical scientist dissolved virtually overnight when he pridefully reported that he had discovered a treat-ment to stave off certain of the ravages of aging, especially those having to do with sexual performance.

Charles-Édouard Brown-Séquard was born in 1817 on the island of Mauritius, to an American father and a French mother. A brilliant researcher, he made many notable contri-butions to the understanding of the nervous system and me-tabolism during his career, and was rewarded by being named professor of experimental physiology at the Collège de France in 1878, in recognition of these and other important ad-vances. He and his predecessor in the college chair, Claude Bernard, are properly credited with introducing the notion that hormones, those protein substances secreted into the bloodstream by ductless glands, control much of the functioning of the internal organs. So impressed was Brown-Séquard by the role of hormones in energizing the animal body and supporting its stability that he began to experiment with them in an effort to rediscover youth.

In 1889, when he was seventy-two years old, Brown-Séquard reported to the French Academy of Sciences that he had been conducting self-experiments in rejuvenation. His method was to crush the testicles of guinea pigs or dogs and innoculate himself with a solution of the fluid thus obtained. Within three days of starting the treatments, he boasted, "I had recovered at least all of my former vigor. . . . My digestion and the working of my bowels have improved considerably too. . . . I also find mental work easier than I have for years." And he added that he had regained his sexual prowess.

Unfortunately, inoculating the same material into others helped no one but Brown-Séquard. The testicular juice may not have helped him very much either, because he died five years later without demonstrating so much as the most minimal objective evidence that he had accomplished anything in the interim except to age in the usual manner of septuagenarians.

Brown-Séquard's attempt to regain his youth became such a target of derision that it besmirched his scientific heritage. But that did not deter others from involving themselves in similar undertakings, whether with testicular or ovarian extracts or the implantation of the organs themselves. Some of the experimenters were established scientists, but others were hucksters in search of a fast buck. A Kansas charlatan named Charles R. Brinkley became wealthy by implanting goats' gonads into many of those suckers who are born every minute, to treat not only aging and impotence but high blood pressure as well. No amount of debunking clamor by physicians or the press in those economically deprived yet in some ways high-flying years of the 1920s and '30s could dim his star, which soared to a height so lofty in the firmament that he eventually ran for governor of his state, electioneering from his own radio station. There is not a shred of evidence that any animal's testicles, ovaries, or similar implanted or injected tissue ever helped so much as a single man or woman to return to youth or sexual potency, nor did it result in other of the consummations devoutly to be wish'd. No one's aging process was halted, and no one became younger.

The reason that Brown-Séquard sometimes enters my thoughts is a memorable conversation I had about six years ago, with a college classmate whom I had not seen in decades. In the midst of the usual comparisons of our former youthful vigor with the current era of rusting joints and battling against the threat of expanding waistlines, he casually dropped the news that he was scheduled to have a penile implant inserted several days hence. A widower of more than a year, he had discovered the tantalizing attractions of much younger women, and found himself sufficiently unpredictable in sexual performance that he was determined to do something about it. Because we were at that time almost half a century out of college, I wondered aloud how many men of our considerable age had undergone such a procedure. My classmate replied that his urologist had assured him that he was far from being the oldest patient in the hospital's surgical series. His next sentence was what started me thinking about Brown-Séquard. "It's not just the sex itself," he said. "It's the feeling that I'm not giving in to old age." It was at this point that I looked more carefully at my erstwhile pal than I had before, and realized that he was wearing a toupee.

A bit later in our brief conversation, he added that he was aware of my having known the man who had invented the device on which he depended to make his sex life so predictable and satisfying. Of course I knew him, and on this hangs, in a manner of speaking, a cautionary tale. The tale, and the caution, are not unrelated to the one my classmate was in the midst of telling me, about the search for evidence of youth not having left the building. Frank Scott, as we called the implant's inventor at the time, was in my class at medical school, and was a notable character even then. I was intrigued by his personality from the start, mostly on account of a unique kind of charisma that I had only read about but until then had never encountered outside of the movies and a few books about the old West. He was a bit over six feet tall and, though somewhat broad-shouldered, was sparely built. Like the cowboy of literature he resembled, Frank was narrow in the waist and hips, and had small but keen eyes that always made him look as though he were peering into a hot sun lying low over the sagebrush, trying to be sure that each of his herd of longhorns was accounted for. Though he came from the city of San Antonio, he wore the aura of all of south-central Texas like a well-fitting ten-gallon hat. If the sum of his appearance did not give away a Lone Star State origin, the drawl certainly did: In general soft and slow, it had a way of sometimes cutting loose like the snap of a whip when he had lost patience with a plodding classmate or an assignment that seemed asinine to him. Of all Frank's characteristics that fascinated me, his ability to turn verbally from the laconic to the fierce and back again in a moment—meantime having struck at his prey like a rattlesnake—was foremost. He had, in addition, a strong-minded Texas self-assurance that some saw as ego. Though usually the most engaging and good-humored of men's men, one could imagine him in another era as a quick and confident gunfighter always ready to draw, striding away after an encounter so that he might finish the job from which he had been momentarily distracted by the nuisance he had just disposed of. Frank Scott always seemed to know what he wanted, and went for it unerringly. He had places to go and things to do, and no patience for delay.

Frank was married to his college classmate, a highly intelligent and prototypically pretty Texas girl named Shirley, who was as patient and gentle as he was unyielding and tough-minded. As did so many other young wives of that era, Shirley put aside her career in order to support her husband's, working at one or another secretarial job at the medical school during their entire four years in New Haven. I don't recall their financial circumstances, but it is hard to believe they were much different from those of almost all the rest of us, who were barely making ends meet in those days of little financial aid or loans. It was a hard life, but most of us somehow thrived on it. The Scotts were doing it together, and even Frank's toughness could not conceal the depth of his love for Shirley, whose life was clearly so wrapped up not only in her adored husband but in his high hopes for the future as well.

In later years, I heard that Frank had gone on to train in urology and eventually become a highly respected professor at the Baylor College of Medicine and the chief of urology at St. Luke's Episcopal Hospital in Houston. And he was the first member of our class to emerge as a well-known medical authority. The reason for the early fame was his invention in 1973 of a device that I can only call "the hydraulic hard-on," to treat the condition nowadays known as erectile dysfunction. Not only had Frank become famous, but he was now rich as well. In addition to having patented his triumph of concept and design and then having founded a company, American Medical Systems—later sold to Pfizer and finally to a group of Wall Street venture capitalists—to develop and manufacture the prosthesis, he had seen to it that no surgeon was permitted to undertake the complex method of inserting it without first passing the expensive instructional course he provided. The money was rolling in—the impotence of other men had made Frank a Texas millionare.

The principle of the hydraulic erection was simple enough, though working out the technical details had been a challenge for a man of Frank's restive nature. The device consists of a small plastic reservoir buried in the fat lying under the skin of the lower abdomen, leading via a narrow tube to two thin-walled flexible cylinders surgically implanted into the penis. When not in use, the cylinders lie empty and flaccid within the normal downward droop of the organ, their presence un-known to any but the informed. But should the urge for coition occur, firm pressure on the reservoir forces its liquid contents into the cylinders, where turgidity is maintained by a system of valves that aids Eros in his work. After consummation has been superseded by afterglow, the cylinders are emptied back into the reservoir by another touch of the fingers, and all is as it was before. Frank's invention of this miracle made instant obsoles-cence of every previous rigid rod of various sorts that had ever been inserted into a recalcitrantly soft penis. The system is on duty at all times, ready to do its libidinal work at a moment's notice. Like my toupeed college chum, thousands—perhaps hundreds of thousands—of men and their consorts have benefited from Frank Scott's ingenuity, and probably his impatience as well. He made it unnecessary to fail, or even to wait.

Frank's invention of the inflatable prosthesis was only one of the many contributions to his specialty for which he became known as one of the most prominent urological innovators of his generation. When he came to our class's twenty-fifth reunion in 1980, he was no longer called Frank, but had become transformed into F. Brantley Scott, now known to his familiars as Brantley. Not only his name was different. Brantley brought with him a perfectly gorgeous woman by all appearances about twenty years younger than he was, whom he introduced as his wife. Shirley, whom so many of us had admired, was in his past. Of all the topics discussed among his classmates on that weekend of alumni nostalgia in early June, the one most commonly mentioned in hushed terms was the transformation of Frank Scott.

Frank's enthusiasm for technology did not end with the innovations he created in the laboratory. He had learned to fly, and a few years after our reunion bought a kit from which he built his own airplane, very likely to make travel easier between Houston and the private island he had bought off the Texas coast. No one will ever know what went wrong on that first test flight, but the craft crashed to the ground with Brantley at the controls. The beautiful young woman was left a widow, and doubtless well provided for. Her husband has since been memorialized as one of the icons of urology, which he certainly was. The department he built at St. Luke's—called

the F. Brantley Scott Department of Urology—is now headed
by the F. Brantley Scott Chair, and the American Foundation
for Urologic Disease each year presents the F. Brantley Scott
Award for Innovation and Creativity in Urology, one of the
specialty's highest honors. As F. Brantley Scott, Frank's heritage added distinction to our medical school class, but those
many of us who liked him so much would prefer to have enjoyed his living presence among our number at each of the
five-year reunions.

Those who find morals in stories such as Frank's will have
good reason to think of the Greek myth of Icarus, who de-
vised feathered wings and attached them to his body with
wax, to help him and his father escape from captivity by
Minos, the Cretan king. According to a standard reference I
have been using for decades, Charles Mills Gayley's 1897 *The
Classic Myths in English Literature,* "Icarus had been warned
not to approach too near to the sun. . . . But then the boy, exulting in his career, soared upward," whereupon the wax
melted and he plunged into a watery grave in the sea beneath.
Frank's innovative use of technology brought him too close
to the sun, some would say. "Exulting in his career" so brilliantly created, he ignored the warnings of others about his
responsibility to those left on the ground who had enabled
the highflier to reach such great heights. This is not to say
that losing his life was the price Frank paid for leaving
Shirley, but the moralists might believe they have good reason
for thinking so. Like my limber college classmate, Frank felt
the need to renew himself. Perhaps his new marriage and
building an airplane were his ways of doing that, just as his
invention of the inflatable prosthesis was the key to my

friend's way of, as he put it, "not giving in to old age." Like everything else about the passing years, these kinds of thing have their plusses and they have their minuses.

Many are the ways of "not giving in to old age," and they have ranged from the pitiably ridiculous to the healthfully sublime. F. Brantley Scott, Charles-Édouard Brown-Séquard, and every hawker of youth-restoring nostrums were appealing to the universal fear of getting old, and to the even greater terror that every evidence of aging brings us further along the road to death. There was general joy a few years ago when molecular biologists began to spread the news that genetic engineering might prove to be the means by which to stave off the inevitable. But that was a mere prelude to the excitement aroused when telomere research was rumored to hold the promise of preventing cells from developing the degenerating changes that gradually cause them to become senile and finally give up their lives. As noted in the previous chapter, scientists are in only the earliest phases of such research, and there is little certainty that it will lead to anything remotely resembling the claims that some have made for it.

Upon hearing word of the new miracles seemingly just beyond the horizon, many a middle-aged man or woman— and no doubt plenty of younger ones too—cuddled up in bed to dream futuristic fantasies. The air became rife (and still is) with possibilities, among which a life span of two or more centuries was not the most extreme. Too few stopped to consider the predictably harmful consequences of such an achievement, not only on human society, but on individuals as well—including those newly spared bicentenarians themselves, cluttering the planet with their needs, their demands, and their refusal to get out of the way. Too few questioned the notion that being able to live a very long time is a good thing—at least for themselves.

From the standpoint of pure biology, we, like all animals, exist in order that we may pass our DNA on to succeeding generations. This is how our species survives; this is how natural selection makes its choices. Once we have lost the ability to reproduce and to nurture our young for a while, we serve no useful function in the grand scheme of nature's relentless events. In the wild, and even among domesticated animals, death shortly after the end of the reproductive years is the rule. Man is one of the few animals to survive much beyond that point. For much of humankind's existence on our planet, in fact, we did not even live long enough to exhaust our reproductive potential. As late as the time of the Roman Empire, when modern *Homo sapiens* had already been in existence for some forty thousand years, average life expectancy was less than thirty years; infectious disease and inadequate nutrition were the big killers, with trauma bringing up the rear. Two millennia later, at the turn of the twentieth century, the life expectancy figure still had not gone much beyond forty-five years, even though most people were far better nourished and more adequately protected from contagion. The average American can mostly thank public health measures such as clean water, immunizations, improved food supply, and good housing for the current expectancy of reaching his or her late seventies. Though the great advances in biomedicine of recent decades have had an effect too—at least in the latter half of the century—only antibiotics and improvements in the treatment of heart disease influence general mortality statistics to a great extent. All the other pharmaceuticals and surgical cobblings affect relatively small numbers of people in the overall figures for the entire world population.

It can never be repeated often enough: Aging is not a disease. It is the condition upon which we have been given life. The aging and eventual death of each of us is as important to the ecosystem of our planet as is the changing of the seasons. Aubrey de Grey prefers to ignore that inconvenient truth, and so do others who applaud his high-wire theoretics. When Dr. William Haseltine, the brilliant biotech entrepreneur who is CEO of the futuristic Human Genome Sciences, Inc., says, "I believe our generation is the first to be able to map a possible route to individual immortality," we should cringe with distaste and even fear, not only at the hubris of such a statement but at its danger to the very concept of what it means to be human. The current biomedical campaign against the natural process of aging is but part of a much larger image of mankind's future, in which it is thought by some to be conceivable that parents may one day order up the IQ, complexion, and stature of their intended offspring, by manipulation of the DNA that goes into their cells. One prophet of unrestrained genetic enhancement, Gregory Stock of Princeton, has gone so far as to entitle his 2002 book about such matters *Redesigning Humans: Our Inevitable Genetic Future* (emphasis mine). Even more frightening than the confidence of Stock's vision for his fellow men and women is the title of the book's first chapter, in which he outlines his notion of how the laboratory will come to control evolution: He calls it "The Last Human," meaning those remaining of us whose bodies and minds have been formed by nature alone. As though to illustrate how palatable these predictions are to those from whom we should have reason to expect a note of caution—who are the putative gatekeepers against such ideas of "progress"—Stock's oeuvre was blurbed by Harold T. Shapiro, once chairman of former president Clinton's National Bioethics Advisory Commission.

These are not the problems with which American medicine or science should be dealing. Their proper task is not the prolongation of life beyond our species's nature-decreed maximum span (which seems to be in the neighborhood of 120 years), but life's betterment. And if anyone's life needs betterment, it is surely the elderly man or woman still living well beyond the years of vigor and productivity because the benisons of public health and biomedicine have made it possible. The percentage of the aged in our population increases with every passing year, and far too many of them are doddering. The very gradual increase in life expectancy of previous generations has been replaced by a surge forward: The twentieth century saw a thirty-three-year gain (more than two years of which came about in the mere decade and a half between 1990 and 2005), an astonishing figure compared to any comparable period in history. Until these recent changes, population size had the general configuration of a pyramid, with a wide base of children, the top narrowing with age. It has now taken on somewhat the shape of a rectangle, as more aged individuals reach the upper levels. As disease treatment continues to improve and public health measures reach a larger segment of the population, this trend will only increase.

Some illustrations provide graphic evidence of these patterns. During the 1990s, the number of American centenarians went from 37,000 to 50,000, and some project that it will reach a million by midcentury. Queen Elizabeth of the United Kingdom customarily sends telegrams to every one of her subjects who attains a hundredth birthday. In the first year of her reign, 1952, the number was 255; it is now well over 5,000. When our nation's Social Security system was established in 1935, it was thought that it would never have to serve more than twenty-five million people. There were more than thirty-eight million beneficiaries in 2000, all but a few million of whom were over sixty-five; it is estimated that the ripening of the baby boomer generation will bring the figure to seventy million by 2011. Nowadays, reaching the once-hoary age of eighty means only that an actuary would predict more than seven years of life remaining. At sixty-five, the figure is almost seventeen years for American men and near twenty for women.

As much as we might hail such statistics, they quite obviously come with a price. Whether the aging process is genetically programmed or results from the gradual wear and tear of a lifetime of internal and external banging around (or, as is most likely, is a combination of both), it is characterized by a journey toward increasing frailty and disability, even for the most robust of the survivors. Joints, bones, hearts, brains, and every other part of us lose their zip, and worse. Many of the 4.5 percent of our population living in long-term-care institutions, and some of those cared for at home, are so incapacitated that they require help with the simplest of needs, like toileting and dressing themselves. Many of them are demented. The number of what geriatricians call "the oldest old"—those over eighty-five—increases with each passing year of improvement in life expectancy. The economic cost is high, but the cost in suffering, not only for the very elderly themselves but for their families, is even greater. For many individuals, the cost of living longer is already too great. Unless major changes are made, the burden on society will become impossible to bear.

And major changes *are* being made. For several decades beyond the time when the nursing homes were beginning to increase in number and the population of frail elderly at home was seen to be rapidly rising, not much progress occurred in ameliorating the conditions faced by old people every day. But the situation began to improve about twenty-five years ago, as more and more studies were undertaken of the factors that determine the disabilities of the aged. At the same time, the still small number of gerontologists—scientists who investigate the process of aging—were increasingly turning their attention toward seeking ways to lessen the ravages of the added years that had been granted to the patients they were studying.

The field underwent a significant philosophical revamping in 1980, when Dr. James Fries, a gerontologist at Stanford University, introduced a concept he called "compression of morbidity." By this, Fries meant the attempt to decrease the period during which any elderly person is disabled. In general, most of us are now fated to endure a final period of years during which we become ever more frail, with the trajectory of decline sloping downward more markedly after the age of around fifty. Fries hypothesized that measures could be taken to change the long, gradually drooping arc with a pattern that more resembled a relatively horizontal line ending in a rapid drop-off shortly before death. If this was accomplished, he pointed out, "then lifetime disability could be compressed into a shorter average period and cumulative lifetime disability could be reduced." In other words, instead of a long period of worsening frailty and illness, our bodies would stay relatively intact and then give out much closer to the time of eventual demise. It is a concept very like the one Oliver Wendell Holmes wrote about in his poem "The Deacon's Masterpiece," in which he describes "the wonderful one-hoss shay, / That ... *breaks down,* but doesn't *wear out.*"

> *You see, of course, if you're not a dunce,*
> *How it went to pieces all at once,—*
> *All at once, and nothing first,—*
> *Just as bubbles do when they burst.*

There are those, of course, who would like to die "all at once," but others would prefer a short period of decline, providing that it is not at all like the agonized waning that so many suffer today. For large numbers of Americans, this is precisely what is already beginning to happen. And there is evidence that such compression of morbidity is within the reach of far more of us.

Among the first steps in the process of change was the realization that physical frailty, and not disease itself or any named pathology, is the most important determinant of whether an elderly person can care for himself and remain a vital contributing member of the community. The older the subject, the more important becomes the role of such factors as muscle strength and bone density, particularly the former. Study after study has confirmed this observation, best stated by a team of gerontologists from the Netherlands in a paper published in *Science* in 1997, as follows: "In the oldest old, loss of muscle strength is the limiting factor for an individual's chances of living an independent life until death." The operative words here are "until death." Before the publication of the Dutch report, and since, repeated studies have shown that feebleness in the elderly not only is preventable but, with an appropriate exercise program, can actually be reversed. Imagine a world in which every very old person might continue to care for himself, enjoy his surroundings, and sustain his loved ones instead of the other way around. And all of this happy state of affairs would go on until near the time of his death.

To the amazement of many a physician who has a large geriatric practice, it has proven to be not difficult to build the necessary muscle, even in the very elderly. It is consistently shown that strength can be almost doubled within six or eight weeks in the oldest old, merely by a supervised regimen of high-intensity resistance training and weights. Though the link between exercise and longevity may no longer be news, only relatively recently has loss of muscle strength been recognized as a major element in causing the disabilities that overtake us as we get older.

In a groundbreaking report published in 1990 in the *Journal of the American Medical Association* and verified by numerous later studies of both men and women, researchers at Tufts University were able to increase the leg muscle strength of ten frail women between the ages of eighty-six and ninety by an average of 174 percent. This was accomplished in a period of eight weeks through a regimen of supervised high-intensity weight training. Although all of the old women in this first study had chronic diseases or disabilities, none of them sustained injuries as a result of the exercises. Their balance improved and so did their walking speed. Among the surprising findings in the many confirmatory studies done since that time is how rapidly the benefits of resistance training become apparent, both by measurements and by improvement in activity.

An example of one of the many supporting studies done subsequent to the Tufts report was one that appeared in February 2006 in the *Journal of Aging and Health*. Gerontologists at the University of South Florida divided a group of sixty-four volunteers with an average age of eighty-four into three groups: no exercise, walking twice a week, and resistance training twice a week. Though generally healthy, some participants needed canes or walkers for their exercise sessions. The results at the end of the sixteen-week study period were not surprising to anyone who had followed the academic literature of geriatrics for the previous decade and a half. The benefits to both categories of exercisers were not confined to improvements in muscle strength. Compared to the inactive group, they had improved not only their upper and lower body strength, but also their performance on tests of agility, balance, and coordination. An added though not entirely unexpected bonus was their lowered systolic blood pressure over the study period. Confirming previous suggestive findings, the researchers pointed out their impression that it may be exercise per se, rather than its type, that results in the observed findings.

But improving muscular power and perhaps other body functions like blood pressure is only part of the answer—the brain needs plenty of attention too. It is by now no secret that continued intellectual stimulation is the key to avoiding many of the ravages of dementia and the apathy that steals the minds of so many institutionalized and homebound elderly. Granted, all the reading and museum-exploring in the world are not likely to reduce the incidence of strokes both large and small, but such activities maintain synapses and probably encourage the development of new brain cells regardless of age. They keep us alert, mentally vital, and curious.

If such factors as vigorous mental and physical exercise have such great benefits for the aged, how much better would the situations of old folks be had they started such exercise far earlier than the period of rapid decline? Though the changes that begin in our late twenties are minimal at first, they speed up after about age thirty, when CT scans actually show evidence of the falling off, such as decreased muscular density and narrower cross-sectional dimensions in the thigh, as well as increasing amounts of fat within individual muscles. Once we reach age fifty, our tendency to dwindle really takes off.

And so, though loss of muscle strength is the limiting factor for the independence of the oldest old, it quite obviously can have profound effects for the rest of us too, and much earlier than most people have realized. But cheer up. As the fitness experts tell us, studies that began with the oldest of the old—those men and women beyond the age of eighty-five— have been extended to younger subjects, with results that are virtually the newest of the new: Such deterioration does not necessarily have to take place. The answer is anaerobic exercise—activity in which the body incurs an oxygen debt. Aerobics—jogging, running on treadmills, pedaling real or stationary bikes, and the like—may do wonders for the heart and lungs, but to ward off feebleness and its associated debility, nothing replaces resistance training with weights. So impressed has the American College of Sports Medicine been by the demonstrable benefits of resistance exercises that it now recommends weight training for all men and women over the age of fifty.

Weight training has yet another advantage over aerobic exercise alone: It uses more calories than such activities as walking, running, or swimming. The reason is that heavy exercise breaks down muscle fibers, whose rebuilding into even greater strength by the body's natural reparative processes requires considerable energy and accordingly burns up lots of calories. On top of that, every new pound of muscle requires thirty to forty calories per day just to maintain it, even when it is at complete rest. So it behooves us all, young or old, to hie ourselves to the nearest gym.

The atmosphere of the typical gym may not at first lend itself to thoughts of mental improvement, but we should think again. Recent studies have found that aerobic fitness in older men and women appears to reduce the loss of brain tissue and improve cerebral functioning. It does this by elevating the levels of brain-derived neurotrophic factor, to which reference was made in chapter 2. BDNF acts to increase the number of synapses, promote the development of new capillaries in the brain, and protect neurons against the damage caused by free radicals. In addition, there is evidence that BDNF may encourage the development of new neurons from adult stem cells. The good news does not end there. Studies done on subjects who have added weight training to aerobic exercise indicate that the combination results in even greater improvement in cognitive functioning than aerobic exercise alone.

Such findings need to be snatched up by all people of all ages. Those of us who are getting on in years, in particular, should snatch them up and run with them—literally. Study after study has shown that exercise of mind and body is the key to increased longevity and prolonged independence. Readers of daily newspapers have seen plenty of reports of leading research groups confirming that vigorous activity in middle-aged or older people prevents or at least significantly lessens loss of muscle strength, which is responsible for so much disability and even disease.

As for intellectual capacity, it has already been pointed out that the best way to maintain mental functioning is to exercise it. The proficiency of the synapse, where an impulse is transmitted from one nerve cell to another, is strengthened by frequent use. The synapse retains its capacity to change, and even to become more effective and stronger, throughout life. This may also be true of the nerve cells themselves. Their ability to generate impulses—what neuroscientists call "electrogenicity"—appears to respond to changes in input. The electrogenic machinery can apparently be remodeled, and patterns of electrical activity altered, depending on the kind and frequency of stimuli that reach the cell. So keep reading this book and plenty of others. You will be strengthening your synapses and building your electrogenicity.

All of this sophisticated talk adds up to no more than the advice that was so often proclaimed by that syndicated sage, the late Ann Landers: "Use it or lose it." And it certainly confirms everyone's daily observations. Simply put, active people remain active. Though it is comforting to have it confirmed by Landers, by laboratories, and by the learned, we have all known for a very long time that the key to productivity is productivity.

What we have not known are the details. At first gradually and now with increasing velocity, not only scientists but fit-

ness experts too are learning the specifics of just what is required to preserve ourselves—if not necessarily to a greater
age, at least to an age less encumbered by the debilities that
too often characterize the final years of life. Even should
"using it" not succeed in prolonging our days, vigorous activity of mind and muscle is the secret of better aging, or what
the gerontologists call "compression of morbidity." The
long-range goal is to make the graph of one's approach to
life's termination cease its agonizingly drawn-out drooping
and come to resemble a vigorous and virtually horizontal line
followed by a more or less perpendicular drop-off.

And as for that end-point date, there is abundant evidence, both anecdotal and statistical, of the beneficial effect
of exercise on life expectancy, and it has been accumulating
for a long time. For example, a long-term evaluation published in 1998 of 52,000 male graduates who entered Har-
vard College and the University of Pennsylvania between
1916 and 1950 showed that alumni between the ages of
thirty-five and seventy-four who over the years expended at
least two thousand calories per week in vigorous activities had
a risk of cardiovascular disease and death that was 25 percent
lower than that of less active men. Not only that, but men
who took up an active life long after college did better than
former student athletes who had quit in middle age. Couch
potatoes should note the jock-image titles of both the article
and the professional publication in which it was printed: "A
Natural History of Athleticism, Health and Longevity," in
the *Journal of Sports Sciences.*

Lest any reader of these pages think I am one of those
above-it-all types who dish out advice and don't take it, I
present here my own personal experience in using the new

knowledge. But first I must point out that I did not go gently. For those unconvinced, reluctant, undecided, or indecisive readers—who, in spite of being much impressed with the findings presented in the foregoing paragraphs are neverthe- less shuffling their feet or thinking, "It's all very well and good for you, Mac, but . . ."—I will simply say that I was once among your number. But I am now a convert and, like so many converts, I have become a zealot. Since the summer of 1998, I have been hauling my aged body off to the gym three times a week, there to sweat among the fit.

No one—but especially no one as predisposed to vanity as a surgeon—would want to be asked by an elder son, "Hey, Pops, wouldn't you like to get some tennis shorts that are a little longer, now that your quads aren't what they used to be?" Coming hard on the heels of a longtime tennis partner's across-the-net observation that "our legs are starting to look as if they belong on a couple of scrawny chickens," the thirty- something's well-intentioned advice was more than a little de- moralizing. I decided then and there that the time had come to pay attention to the repeated urgings (truth to tell, they were more like hectorings) of my wife, who had been looking svelter by the week as the result of rising at five o'clock each morning to pump iron, go spinning, and run stationary laps at a local gym.

Within days, I had signed up for an exercise program at a facility a few miles from my home, called—what else?—the In Shape Fitness Center. Being committed to the principle that all novitiates need a role model, I found myself a deceptively sweet-natured Atlas of a trainer named Dave Butler, and told him that I wanted to be just like him when I grew up. Gra- ciously ignoring the fact that I am thirty-five years older than he, my new mentor took me at my word. Aware that it was far too late to acquire a sweet nature, I nevertheless did harbor an aging male's fantasy about emulating Dave's strength. But first, my immediate goal was to get the old legs back and flatten a gut that was just beginning to make itself evident.

Dave took a long list of measurements, made a series of calculations, and set up a program of resistance training and cardiovascular exercise. It wasn't a menu for the faint of heart, and in spite of his gentle demeanor, Dave proved to be a young man of forceful determination, setting me loose in the gym on my own with the admonition that he expected real improvement by the time we met again in six weeks.

In matters like these, it helps to have a compulsive personality, and that is where the three decades in the operating room paid off. I have been religious about my exercise routine, both during those initial six weeks and since. What do I care that just about every other male in the gym is in his twenties or thirties and is pumping as much as twice the iron that I do? And why be concerned that more than a few times I have followed a twenty-one-year-old coed onto a machine and had to remove thirty or forty pounds from the weight pile before lifting?

The first of my rewards came when Dave did his second set of calculations at the six-week mark, and the rewards have continued. In my initial eight months of sweating and straining, I took off nine pounds of fat and added six pounds of muscle mass. My waist was two inches narrower than before and my chest an inch and a half wider. The percentage of my body that was fat had dropped from 21 (in the range called "acceptable" on the fitness charts) to 16 (in the middle of the category designated as fit/healthy). The improvements had come about without an iota's change in my eating habits, although Dave originally outlined a nutrition plan that I had gleefully ignored. I was, in fact, In Shape. I found myself able to run around a tennis court as I had not since my thirties. On my son's next visit, I put on (short) bathing trunks, in order to show off my newly sculpted chest and abdominal muscles, which by then I had taken to calling pecs and abs. An unexpected dividend was that many of the little muscular aches and pains to which we senior citizens force ourselves to become inured had either disappeared or lessened.

But I have to confess to a couple of disappointments. It is claimed that consistent exercise lowers cholesterol, and so I followed its blood level periodically for some time. After a small initial drop, it went right back to its previous high, and it has stayed there. And then there was the testosterone story. I had read reports that its concentration rises with anaerobic exertion, and mine did in fact shoot up to a stratospheric level by the four-month mark and continued to rise afterward. With testosterone like that, I should have been bounding around like a satyr chasing nymphs. When I noticed no change in my amatory inclinations, I queried a friend who specializes in knowing a thing or two about hormones. He gently broke the sad news that heavy exercise increases the secretion of a protein that binds testosterone, which is why its blood level rises. But a bound testosterone molecule is like a bound stallion—it can't run with the herd. It's the *free* testosterone that does the real job, and mine had gone up less than 10 percent. And so, the nymphs were safe and I've never tested my blood level of male hormone again.

Here it is necessary to state the obvious. It is clear from this description that my motivation to join the gym had little to do with health per se, and everything to do with vanity. But it hardly makes a whit of difference. The magnet may be the means, but the real object is the outcome. Vanity has its uses, and among them is that ages-old urge that drew Brown-Séquard to his guinea pig gonads and me to my machines. For me, the result of all the years of sweating and straining has been mobility, coordination, strength, weight control, and a sense of pride that buoys me up each time I think about what has been accomplished by sticking to my resolve. And for all I know, the increased BDNF has all the time been doing wonders for my synapses and neurons. And there are all those studies I read about in my medical journals, telling me that there is now statistical evidence that psychological depression is decreased in frequency and degree by vigorous exercise, and the likelihood of certain forms of cancer is lessened. These are bonuses I had not expected when I began on that summer afternoon in 1998, but I accept them willingly. There is a thin and very indistinct line that separates a man's vanity from his pride—and a woman's too, I would guess—and I don't really care which side of it I stand on, so long as it keeps me in the gym, which I have come to think of as essential to my well-being.

Because the benefits of vigorous activity as well as other remedies such as cessation of smoking, proper diet, and certain medical means (daily vitamins, calcium supplements, and perhaps a baby aspirin, for example) have been known for decades and have been adhered to by millions of Americans, these benefits should by now be measurable statistically. Have the benefits, in fact, resulted in compression of morbidity? Evidence from a series of surveys in which researchers followed older adults from 1982 until 1999 indicates that they have. An article published in the *Journal of the American Medical Association* in December 2002 reports that physical, cognitive, and sensory limitations in those who are vigorously active are beginning to decrease. Not only that, but the proportion of people over the age of sixty-five living in institutions for the debilitated elderly has dropped from 6.3 percent to 4.5 percent during the seventeen years of the studies. There are plenty of journal publications demonstrating similar results, including a well-known one in which a large group of University of Pennsylvania alumni averaging sixty-eight years of age at the beginning of the study were found to have postponed disability by an average of 7.75 years if they exercised, avoided cigarettes, and had normal body mass, compared to their counterparts who did not.

As so frequently happens when changes in large populations are studied, the statisticians have the last word. In the case of the elderly, they have expressed it most recently in a United States government report issued jointly by the Department of Health and Human Services and the Department of Commerce, entitled *65+ in the United States: 2005*. Published in December of that year, the report utilizes information garnered by the Census Bureau to present an overview of both the current and coming elderly American population, which can be extrapolated, it is probably safe to say, to most industrialized nations of the world.

The entire report can be epitomized by a single sentence that appears on its very first page: "The older population is on the threshold of a boom." By this is meant not only a boom in numbers but a boom in health, education, prosperity, and even optimism. And as is obvious to any but the most superficial observers of the present-day scene, the boom has been under way for some time. In fact, the word "boom" would seem to be particularly appropriate, since the proximate cause of some of the increase in numbers is the graying of the baby boomers, a generation that began its existence in 1946. The health and socioeconomic profile of the average older American of today is markedly different from that of his or her predecessor in earlier generations, and it will be even more so as the coming decades arrive. Though most of the information in 65+ *in the United States: 2005* deals with length of life, it is sprinkled throughout with evidence of life's increasing quality as well.

According to the report, the number of Americans over sixty-five is projected to be 72 million by 2030 (nearly 20 percent of the population at that time) and 86.7 million in 2050, as compared to 36 million in 2003. Even without boomers, the number of the oldest old has also been growing rapidly, already being 4.7 million in 2003, projected to almost 10 million in 2030 and 21 million in 2050. Much the same can be said of centenarians, whose number, as already noted, has already gone from about 37,000 in 1990 to 50,000 in 2000. At present, 64 percent of Americans can expect to live to at least seventy-five, and 35 percent to at least eighty-five. Not only that, but the number of years of remaining life expectancy is also going up for all of the elderly. The average seventy-five-year-old American man of today can anticipate more than another ten years on this earth, while his twin sister will be around for more than twelve.

The growth in size of the population that is sixty-five and older is far outpacing that of people younger than that age, and at present accounts for one in eight Americans. All of this reflects, of course, increases in the average life expectancy, which has gone from 47.3 years in 1900 to an average of 77.9 years in 2004, meaning that the average girl born in that year will live to be eighty, and the average boy to seventy-five. Much of the change has been due (and this is remarkably different from the cause of earlier increases, which were in greatest part due to lessened mortality among infants and the young) to reductions in mortality among the elderly population.

These numbers are abetted by the fact that the first of the baby boomers will turn sixty-five in 2011, but that cohort is far from the numbers' entire basis. In the words of the report, "People in the United States are living longer and healthier lives than ever before." The frequency and mortality of the leading killer, heart disease, continues to drop; this decline is, in fact, the most important reason for the overall decline in death rates among the elderly. Moreover, studies of the type described in the previous pages of this book reveal considerable decline in rates of general disability and in limitations of functioning. "In order to address quality of life, the concept of active life expectancy (ALE) is used to measure the number of years that people can expect to live on an average without disability. Using various measurements and methods of analysis, including ALE, recent studies conclude that in addition to living longer, the current generation of older people are [sic] healthier and less disabled than their predecessors."

These changes are due to such factors as higher socioeconomic status and net worth (for example: 35 percent of the elderly population lived below the poverty line in 1959, as compared to 10 percent by 2003. Moreover, the median household income in homes with a householder over sixty-five has risen from $12,882 in 1967 to $23,787 in 2003, adjusted for inflation); improved diet (due to such factors as higher standards of living as reflected in income, better education, and increased knowledge of nutrition both by medical science and the general population); more understanding of the importance of physical and intellectual activity and other positive behavioral changes; decreased smoking (cigarettes are more dangerous for the elderly than for younger smokers, not only because they add to pathology already made significant by long-standing addiction to nicotine, but also on account of cigarettes' effect on the chronic diseases so often found among older people); and continuing scientific research on the biology and medical consequences of aging. As noted earlier, by far the most important factor in increasing longevity and general vitality during the first half of the twentieth century was improvements in the public health by such means as immunizations, water purification, more adequate housing, better clothing, and enhanced sanitation. During more recent decades, medical progress benefiting individual patients has become a bigger factor and holds the promise of more effective treatment for cancer, lung disease, stroke, and such chronic debilitating diseases as diabetes, hypertension, osteoporosis, kidney failure, Alzheimer's and other dementias, and arthritis. The campaign against chronic disease is particularly important for quality of life, because about 80 percent of the elderly have at least one chronic health condition and 50 percent have at least two.

Factors other than healthful lifestyles and improved attention to fitness have quite obviously contributed to these salutory statistics. Nevertheless, there can be little doubt that relatively simple measures to encourage these two factors, such as those being recommended by gerontologists and their clinical colleagues, the geriatricians, play a major role in their attainment. There is reason for optimism in these figures, and hope that in future decades even fewer of our nation's elderly will be confined to nursing homes or will be dependent on others for the needs of daily living.

In a time of finite resources—and when have we lived in a time when resources were not finite?—we would do well to expend far more of our intellectual and fiscal capital on improving the quality of our later lives than on the self-absorbed and very likely fanciful goal of lengthening our lives beyond that 120 years allotted by natural selection. An enlarging pool of the elderly have much to offer our society, if we can but help them to remain sufficiently vital to bring their potential benefits to the rest of us. Instead of spending vast amounts of money on today's version of Brown-Séquard's fantasy—rejuvenation clinics, where hormones and fetal cells are injected, and fistfuls of antioxidants are swallowed—instead of spending vast amounts of money supporting eager scientists who promise life everlasting by molecular sleight-of-hand—instead of such folly, we should look at the aged among us and realize their need, and ours.

Some of those aged are already showing us the potential value of such investments in the quality of their lives. The compressed morbidity and postponement of disability that has benefited so many of them—as well as the increased longevity—are becoming enough that we see examples of it every day. A mere look around us confirms those statistical studies that give scientific objectivity to a phenomenon visible to anyone who thinks about it. The older men and women we encounter as we go about our daily routines do look and act much younger than their predecessors did a generation ago.

And we see far more instances of individuals whose lives are in many respects just as useful to society and rewarding to themselves as they were at the height of their working careers. They exemplify what could be done, if only the knowledge and the resources were made available to everyone.

Emanuel Papper, who died at the age of eighty-seven in December 2002, was my closest and most admired friend. An air force medical officer decorated with the Silver Star for heroism, he emerged from World War II with internal injuries to the diaphragm and stomach sustained when his bomber was shot down, and from which he never fully recovered. Realizing that the field of anesthesiology was still in a relatively primitive state, he determined to do something about it. He was able to accomplish his goal by introducing the principles of basic science research into clinical care and the training of residents, an approach that he and only a few other pioneers brought to academic medical centers in the 1950s. As chairman of the department of anesthesiology at his alma mater, Columbia University, he organized a program that attracted colleagues from all over the world, who came to learn his methods and bring them back to their own hospitals and medical schools.

After twenty-five years of directing one of America's premier departments in his specialty, Manny Papper accepted the position of dean of the medical school at the University of Miami. His tenure there lasted fourteen years, during which he made vast improvements in the institution's academic standards before retiring at the age of seventy. Though he continued to teach residents and students in anesthesiology, his inquiring mind demanded new challenges, and he enrolled in the university's doctoral program in English literature, and was awarded his Ph.D. degree when he was seventy-six. The dissertation he wrote on the Romantic poets provided grist for his multi-focused intellectual mill for the rest of his life, and he continued to pore over the works of early-nineteenth-century authors and to acquire first editions of their works for his increasingly formidable collection. His intellectual interests were broad, including the study of religions, classical music, the masterpieces of painting of virtually every style, and a great curiosity about the undertakings of the wide variety of men and women with whom he came into contact.

Though essentially living a life of the mind, Manny Papper never neglected his body. He exercised regularly and strenuously, and was an avid tennis player until only a few years before his death. Anyone traveling to visit him in Miami was likely to be taken to the gym, and later invited to join him on one of his long, vigorous walks, which tired many a younger man or woman before their host was noticeably affected.

As Manny approached his middle eighties, he gradually developed shortness of breath and began to become more easily fatigued than he had previously. A major abdominal operation to treat a life-threatening emergency caused by the old war wounds added to the magnitude of these problems, but he recovered rapidly and resumed his usual program of exercise, never having slackened off in his intellectual pursuits. When medical evaluation showed the breathing difficulties to be the consequence of a leaking heart valve, he resolved to undergo the hazardous surgery that would be required to repair it, because the respiratory limitations had begun to infringe on his enjoyment of life, which still included a regimen of weight training and walking, though he had reluctantly abandoned tennis a few years earlier due to a shoulder injury.

The events of September 11, 2001, reignited Manny's long-standing interest in Islam, which he began to study with the same intensity that he had always applied to every other of his pursuits, going so far as to organize a conference on the subject at the Aspen Institute, of whose board he was a member of long standing. Late one afternoon in early December 2002—a few weeks before the scheduled heart surgery—while exploring the Internet in hope of finding the answer to some abstruse problem in Islamic history, Manny suddenly complained of blurriness of vision, and then fell unconscious to the floor. He died in the hospital seven hours later, of a massive cerebral hemorrhage.

Of course, the story of Manny Papper represents an extreme example of what is possible, given the will and the wherewithal. He had the background, the personal drive, and the financial resources to live his years in a way that fulfilled his greatest hopes. But the important lesson to be learned from his tale's telling is that this kind of thing is possible, even if not very often to the extent that he was able to enjoy. What is required is for the public to understand the rather simple principles that prevent disability while increasing the quality of life, and probably its quantity as well. And what is also needed is continued intensive research into the causes of disability, which would encourage prevention by the aging themselves, a category that each of us joins the moment we leave the womb. Better to spend our nation's money in such ways than to waste it in the vainglorious search for immortality.

And if a few of our elder citizens believe that a more

youthful outlook is attained by wearing a toupee or a wig, it is not for the rest of us to ridicule. Instead, we should consider that such stratagems are only a manifestation of the wish to remain young, and are perhaps the first step toward changing the long-standing self-destructive habits and buying the gym membership that will really do the job. Vanity is like the raisins that draw a kid to the cereal, and pride is the richness of flavor that keeps him eating it. And as for the penile implant that my former classmate is planning: Am I the only old codger who is beginning to think that it may not be such a bad idea after all?

NINE

WISDOM, EQUANIMITY, CARING— PRINCIPLES FOR EVERY AGE

I n a book on aging, it would seem a worthy undertaking to reflect on wisdom. And so, as a man of now considerable years and therefore some prerogative, I will not hesitate to do just that, accompanied by the hope that I can avoid the great temptation of waxing ponderous.

Every culture associates being wise with older people, though it is well known that merely being old does not in itself confer wisdom, nor does being young prevent it. Plenty of elders have never achieved it, perhaps most. And plenty of elders are foolish, even long before they become senile. If we are to extract wisdom from our years as they are being lived, we must begin early to acquaint ourselves with wisdom's qualities, and absorb them into all that we are trying to become.

Like aging itself, the having of wisdom is a stage of ongoing development, whose degree of success depends upon every other stage that came before it. Because its evolution in any individual ordinarily requires the long passage of time, it is in general safe to say that seniors are more likely to be wise than their juniors, though an abundance of exceptions do occur among the young. Whatever its degree of justification, the belief that wisdom is the province of age is reflected in many cultures, but in no language more directly than in Hebrew, where the word for "old," *zaken,* is an acronym formed from the expression, *zeh kanah hokhmah,* literally "this one has acquired wisdom."

Though age may not necessarily bring wisdom, age nevertheless demands it. At earlier stages of our lives, things tend to take care of themselves. They do not require the consistent attention and watchful circumspection we come to need in order to negotiate our later decades. When we are young, errors are more easily retrieved and false steps more easily retaken. As we age, we must learn to do without the second or third chances and the compensatory readjustments that have worked so well in the past to maintain the balance and forward motion of our lives. As Michael DeBakey would surely point out, we can replace the automatically stabilizing gyroscope with wisdom, if we have it. But we will not have it if we assume that it is necessarily the reward of age, without our having prepared for it—without our having accumulated it along the way. We are aided in wisdom's pursuit by the length of our days, but our days must have been well used in the decades before they have grown long.

Asked to designate the most direct path toward wisdom, I would unhesitatingly point to the conscious and unconscious modeling of ourselves on those whom we believe wise. Who among us has not more than once approached a vexing problem by thinking back on how it might have been solved by someone whose judgment we have admired and attempted to emulate? We come to recognize such men and women when we encounter them, just as we recognize wisdom from whatever source it may spring.

It is wise also to learn from exemplars of the past. We study history, wrote Sir William Osler, the first professor of medicine at Johns Hopkins University, "for the silent influence of character on character." But it is in the ordinary course of our daily lives that the wise are most usefully encountered, sometimes in the most unlikely places and among the most unlikely kinds of people. We should be constantly on watch for them, and pay attention. "Wisdom is the reward you get," Mark Twain is reputed to have said, for once without tongue in cheek, "for a lifetime of listening when you would rather have talked." Though the unassailably perfect wise man does not exist, the continuum of wisdom is everywhere around us.

The getting of wisdom is, of course, a process, and it has no end point. There is no recognizable peak on which the seeker may finally stand and say, "Now I am wise." The process is incomplete at any stage, and the outcome, like all good, is relative.

The wisdom that we seek with age is not something that comes without effort, nor is it unearned consolation for the passage of years. Rather, it is the result of reflecting. As we grow older, an appreciation for the value of unhurried judgment and the careful weighing of long-term consequences expands. If the aging brain is well used, knowledge grows as does the inclination and the opportunity to integrate knowledge into reflective thought.

We tend to call someone wise if he or she consistently

makes good decisions and knows how to help others do the same. But these are only *manifestations* of wisdom, its outward evidence. They tell nothing of its components and the basis upon which wise people incorporate those components into their own character and behavior. Everything that follows here is based on a single proposition: The wise man or woman strives to know how the moral, useful, and rewarding life should be lived—and lives it. To know it without living it is to be a head without a body.

Knowledge is not wisdom. Wisdom involves the *management* of knowledge, which in turn involves comprehension of the significance of the knowledge possessed. Wisdom is knowledge put to use by judgment. T. S. Eliot expressed his understanding of this in his pageant play, *The Rock*:

> *Where is the wisdom we have lost in knowledge?*
> *Where is the knowledge we have lost in information?*

Of the many kinds of knowledge upon which wisdom is based, the foremost must surely be *self*-knowledge, hard-won and often difficult to face. As more than one wag has put it, "The trouble with self-knowledge is that it's so often bad news." Bad news or not, it must be dealt with. Like no other characteristic of wisdom, this one is elusive, and too often the very thing we try so hard to avoid. The self-knowledge we believe ourselves to possess may actually be the self-delusion behind which we hide. But we fool ourselves at our own peril, and the peril only increases as we age. The slightest admission to one's conscience of such a truth is the beginning of self-knowledge and well worth the pursuing, difficult though it may be.

In the *Dialogues of Plato,* we read, "For self-knowledge would certainly be maintained by me to be the very essence of knowledge, and in this I agree with him who dedicated the inscription, 'Know thyself!' at Delphi." To know oneself is to recognize and acknowledge insecurities, fears, biases, ambition, competitiveness—and hopes, too. For these are the influences that have the potential to distort the clarity of mind, purpose, and motivation so urgently needed if proper judgments are to be reached.

Motive lies behind every decision we make, and it is never pure. In the interest of judicious precision of thought, the nature and content of mixed motive must be known so well and confronted so honestly that it is not allowed to distract from the calculus of reasoning. Accustomed as we are to scrutinizing the motives of others, it is incumbent on us—more than incumbent, it is an urgent necessity—that we scrutinize our own. In the words of Marcus Aurelius, "Accustom yourself in the case of whatever is done by anyone, so far as possible to inquire within yourself: 'To what end does this man do this?' And begin with yourself and first examine yourself." When we are sufficiently familiar with the world within us, we perceive why we are inclined to respond as we do to the world around us, and are in this way equipped to make choices about our appropriateness of response in any given situation.

To know oneself is also to know the limits of one's knowledge, to accept them if they cannot be changed, and to take that into consideration in the same way that motive is taken into consideration. How many of us are willing to look at the limits of our knowledge and take account of them? Here follows the narrative of a man whose career's greatest contribution was based on the enviable characteristic of having that particular component of wisdom, though he may have had no other. Not only was he wise in this one thing, but his example taught others, in accordance with the general principle that we must seek wisdom anywhere it can be found, even at the unlikeliest of sources. In the "Pirke Avoth"—Ethics of the Fathers—in the Talmud, Rabbi Ben Zoma asks, "Who is wise?" And then answers his own question by saying, "He who learns from all men."

At the hospital then called Grace–New Haven, he was listed in the directory of physicians as James P. Mignone, Jr., M.D. But I never heard him referred to as Dr. Mignone unless he was right there to hear it, and even his colleagues did not call him Jim except when speaking directly to him. Out of his immediate earshot, he was invariably called Jimmymignone— not Jimmy, not Mignone, and certainly not *Dr.,* but always the whole thing pronounced quickly without pause as if it were one word—and it seemed to fit his hurried ways perfectly. Our senior professors used that sobriquet when speaking of him, whether to medical students or to the hospital barber. Even to some of our barely literate cafeteria workers back then in the 1950s, he was Jimmymignone. From the loftiest to the lowliest, he was what he was.

What he was was the family physician to the Family. Jimmymignone was New Haven's Mafia doctor. Rumor had it that the New England mob was then run by a godfather in Providence, and our small city of about 150,000 was the second most important crime town in the entire region. Not Boston, not Bangor, and not even Bridgeport, but New Haven, Connecticut. It was an honor of sorts, I suppose, and we medical students treated Jimmymignone with a certain modicum of what I can only call awe. We were more impressed than amused by his ability to, while in the middle of one of his typical rapid-fire sentences, turn suddenly on his heel in such a swift flash of movement that we more often than not found ourselves cut off without being able to respond. We would then be left staring at the receding sight of the pin-striped back of his expensive double-breasted suit as he raced up the corridor.

All of Jimmymignone's movements were quick. He made rounds on his many hospitalized patients each morning with the alacrity of a terrier trying to outrun the dog warden. Looking down on the doctors' parking lot from a height of seven stories, we would sometimes see him scurry across the pavement to his shiny Cadillac and then roar off to the other hospital in the city, or—in our imaginations—to a don's behind-the-pizzeria office, to scribble one of the narcotic prescriptions because of which he was so often in trouble with the New Haven police, or at least those few cops who were not part of his circle. In reality, the reason for his haste was simply that he had to get back across town to see the office full of patients always waiting for him there. Jimmymignone had the largest medical practice in New Haven.

Jimmymignone was a nice guy. His natural affability and New Haven's then-large population of Italian-born immigrants made him a much sought-after physician, and he refused his services to no one, even though they might be unable to pay. He was not the Mafia doctor for any nefarious reason, but simply because the mobsters liked him and he was never unavailable to them or anyone else in medical need. I always suspected that his excessive narcotic-prescribing was due more to his inability to refuse anyone—including mafiosi—than to a thirst for ill-gotten gain. In return, the mobsters used their connections to help him avoid prosecution, and the cops were reluctant to punish a man they admired.

Jimmymignone was always smiling. I never saw him without a wide grin on his olive-complected, hawk-nosed visage. No single slick of his thinning black hair was anything but flatly combed directly backward on his long narrow head. He looked like a happy blackjack dealer. Jimmymignone grinned so much not only because of his basically sunny nature but also because he wanted to be sure of the good will of the interns and residents. When I knew him, he was in his late fifties, having obtained his medical degree three decades earlier as one of the many American students then enrolled at the University of Bologna, a once-distinguished institution then in a long period of decline from which it has since brilliantly recovered. To no one's recollection had he ever written an order in a chart.

Though Jimmymignone had plenty of patients in the hospital at any given time, he didn't actually take care of them, because he did not know how. Any medical problem not of a magnitude to be handled quickly in an office setting was beyond him, and he made no pretensions otherwise. The result was that his inpatients were very carefully watched over by the interns, residents, and attending physicians on the medical school faculty. Because everyone liked Jimmymignone and everyone knew how clinically inept he was, a kindly conspiracy of nurture existed around him and around each of his patients. The result was excellent medical care.

Among wisdom's various components, none are thought by most people to be more important than length of time on this earth and the experiences through which one has lived.

Jimmymignone had more medical experience than any doctor I knew in those days, and yet he was one of the least able. Though he treated so many men and women in his office, and saw how they were cared for in the hospital, he was unable to reflect on any of that, or to gain from it in a way that approximated, at least to us students, medical wisdom. His original base of knowledge was poor. That and his nonreflective turn of mind prevented him from utilizing what passed before his eyes every day; he was immune to improving himself. As one of my teachers once said, "If time and experience were what counted most, Jimmymignone would be the best clinical physician in the state, but he's probably one of the worst, at least from the standpoint of diagnosis and therapy."

But Jimmymignone was blessed with that quality too often disregarded when wisdom is considered. Though he knew so little of clinical medicine, his great strength was *self-*knowledge. He knew his limits and he used that awareness to do well by the people who entrusted themselves to him. He did only what he was qualified to do, and saw to it that others more skilled took over where his abilities left off. In this he was wise, because his patients always got the best possible care. And so in the end, who is to say that Jimmymignone was not a good doctor? And who is to say he was not a wise man? And who is to say that he was not someone from whom the rest of us could learn something important?

I have been writing here of self-knowledge as though it is attainable in all of its dimensions. But the truth is somewhat different. Like wisdom itself, self-knowledge can only be approached but never fully achieved. By introspection, brutal honesty, and the capacity to acknowledge any questionable inclinations, it is possible to come closer to the desired goal.

Though wisdom involves the search for ultimate truth, it must be pursued with the realization that ultimately there is no absolute truth, only perception. Ambiguity, contradiction, uncertainty, even error: To be comfortable with them is the beginning of wisdom. To function and make good decisions in the face of uncertainty, unpredictability, and necessarily limited information is to acknowledge that these are intrinsic to the human condition, the conditions of our lives. To deal with them requires flexibility, and this too is a component of wisdom. To step back, constantly reevaluate, modify judgments, and be willing to admit inaccuracy and error—these test wisdom's resolve.

Wisdom has a purpose; that purpose is action. This means that action must sometimes be taken with the full understanding that decisions may possibly result in less than perfect consequences. Because taking action in the face of incomplete information is the usual condition in which wisdom needs to be applied, each choice, no matter how wise and with what good outcome, is a choice likely to have some drawbacks of its own, just as even wonder drugs have side effects of which account must be taken in their use. It is in weighing what might be called the cost-benefit ratio of each decision that wisdom faces one of its most difficult tests. Knowing that unwelcome imperfections are the inevitable accompaniments of even the wisest decisions should never paralyze decision-making, or cause hesitancy in a decision's implementation. The wise take action in the face of imperfect knowledge, and even given the probability of imperfect solutions.

It is for such reasons that the wise are characterized by their ability to anticipate the consequences of the choices they make. While such foresight requires a richness and variety of life's previous experience, even more important is the ability to interpret that experience, to mine it for meaning. Those who have delved deeply are equipped to recognize patterns that will likely play themselves out when certain courses of action are taken. This connecting of the past with the present and future—for which older men and women are well suited—may not guarantee unfailingly accurate prediction in all cases, but it does allow the envisioning of a trajectory on which any given decision most probably will project itself.

This enables what is called "intuition," which is nothing more than the harvest of that constant processing of information going on within the mind, often below the level of knowing thought. The so-called intuition of the wise is hard-bought, and it comes from the synthesis of a long experience of experiences, and the capacity to organize these experiences into a coherent system of patterns and priorities that is stored in the brain's memory banks, ever ready to be called on as circumstances demand. We are made of memories; the structure and condition of our lives at any moment is in large part the consequence of every decision we have made until that time. An ethic of personal responsibility for those decisions and the actions that have followed from them is the province of the wise.

The wise learn equally from the good and bad, success and failure; they live through hard times and tragedy, and use them for the lessons such times can teach. In tragedy, the unwise see only loss; the wise find meaning. Many of us, in fact, are far better at learning from tragedy than from great good fortune, which we somehow regard as mere luck, without stopping to consider the elements of it in which we may have had a hand or which may be useful for future decision-making. Think here of the philosophy of Miriam Gabler, as expressed in the epigraph of chapter 4.

In all of these considerations, the wise deal with the world as it really is; they do not create scenarios to serve some desired purpose. To be wise is to abjure self-delusion—to see things, including ourselves, as they are, while retaining the optimism to see them as we hope they can be. The wise man or woman is both a dreamer and a person of action, at once an idealist and a realist, a visionary with feet sturdily planted in the terra firma of here and now.

To see the world as it really is demands a certain degree of objectivity, even detachment—but never aloofness. One's own needs, feelings, or emotions must be taken into consideration, but they should not be allowed to color judgment insofar as such a thing is humanly possible. In other words, the approach to judgment and knowledge should be so reflective that it transcends one's personal concerns and self, aiming instead for the humanistic, even the universal. It is the human condition that motivates the wise, rather than their place in it.

The notion of the human condition refers to individuals more than to a general state of the mass of mankind. Accordingly, the ultimate concern of the wise should first be for the welfare of individuals, and only then extending on a gradual continuum to the families, groups, and societies of which they are a part.

Obligation to distinct people would seem to be at odds

with an attitude of detachment, especially when this obligation includes allowing oneself to take an interest in those people, even feeling a closeness toward them. We cannot take responsibility for one or several others without having personal feelings for them. Responsibility involves dedication, a mere step from devotion.

The single word that best incorporates what I am trying to communicate here is "caring." Caring arises from an inner sense of relatedness to one or more individuals and to all humankind, and the recognition that humankind's ultimate good is bound up with one's own. Caring has about it something of the nature of wonder, that one's own strivings can be transcended in the name of a greater principle, one that ultimately benefits everyone.

This is precisely what Saint Paul must have meant by the ringing words of chapter 13 in I Corinthians, when he said that *agapé,* in the original Greek, is greater even than faith and hope. *Agapé* refers to a kind of wondrous love, which the authors of the Vulgate properly translated into the Latin *caritas,* best defined as a "caring love" that puts aside petty self-interest. Saint Paul's magnificent words epitomize much of what has already appeared in the present and earlier chapters of this book: "And now abideth faith, hope and *caritas,* these three; but the greatest of these is *caritas.*" Where there is no *caritas,* there can be no wisdom.

If there is no *caritas* for others as individuals and in the aggregate, wisdom cannot survive. But few of us have been endowed with enough of it by nature or nurture, and fewer still have been able to retain what we have of it through a lifetime of the realities in daily experience and the cynicism these realities often engender. Concern for others is viewed by some as a theoretical virtue toward which there is no easy or even discernible path. But plenty of men and women before us have tried to point the way. Percy Shelley, one of those precociously wise young people—those exceptions—of whom note was taken at the beginning of this chapter, mused at the age of twenty-seven on a quality that might be called "moral imagination," and in his essay "A Defence of Poetry" he told how it could be achieved.

> The great secret of morals is love; or a going out of our own nature, and an identification of ourselves with the beautiful which exists in thought, action, or person, not our own. A man, to be greatly good, must imagine intensely and comprehensively; he must put himself in the place of another and of many others; the pains and pleasures of his species must become his own. The great instrument of moral good is the imagination.

The putting of ourselves "in the place of another and of many others" is a road toward *caritas* well worth the traveling. We nowadays call it "empathy," but perhaps it can mean a little more than that; perhaps it can mean to imagine not only seeing the world through the eyes and feelings of others but more specifically seeing *ourselves* that way—to look into the eyes of another and see ourselves reflected there; to live up to the best expectations of those closest to us, and by such means come nearer to *caritas,* to mature reflection, and to principled living. To be wise, one must first be good.

To deal with such complexities requires equanimity, the acquired talent of being imperturbable, defined by William Osler in 1889 as "presence of mind under all circumstances, calmness amid storm, clearness of judgment in moments of grave peril," and elsewhere by him as "firmness and courage, without, at the same time, hardening 'the human heart by which we live.' . . . How difficult to attain, yet how necessary, in success as in failure!"

Real imperturbability is, in fact, so difficult to attain that it is beyond the reach of most—and perhaps all—of us, in addition to being one of those several qualities that exist as a matter of degree rather than complete achievement: In any given situation of stress, there is some greater or lesser element of perturbation; one would have to be an inhuman paragon not to feel it. More important than being imperturbable, therefore, is the way we deal with stress. When we admit to ourselves that we are anxious, and understand that it is the natural outgrowth of the particular situation we are in, such an acknowledgment renders it more acceptable to us and makes it less likely that we will think ourselves inadequate for feeling it. The result is a lessening of anxiety's hold, sometimes just enough to help with the clarity of thinking that permits finding a way out of the difficulty being faced.

In a long surgical career, I have found myself terrified—scared out of my wits—in the operating room on about four or five occasions. Each time, it was because a sudden and life-threatening hemorrhage of high-pressure arterial blood had occurred under circumstances so unforeseeable that I was completely unprepared for the possibility that it might happen. A surgeon is faced with massive blood loss frequently, but the only times I ever felt this sort of fear were when I thought it had been caused by my own error, as by overly hasty dissection, clumsiness, or some similar inadequacy. What saved me—and the patient—when these episodes occurred was my years of residency training, during which I had occasionally seen some of my most respected teachers get into this kind of trouble. As a result, I could summon the emotional wherewithal to immediately forgive myself when such things happened to me, rather than giving in to the intense self-reproach that might stand in the way of doing what was instantaneously needed in order to get out of the desperate difficulties engendered by my own hands. If the finest of my mentors had had such problems, I could hardly condemn myself.

During those many years of surgery, I had a whole catalogue of ways to restore equanimity when it threatened to leave me. Perhaps there are lessons in them that might be generally useful to others as well for the kinds of agitations that threaten the calm so badly needed to make good decisions under extreme stress. Humor, even clumsy humor, helped. On more than one occasion when immersed in a dissection so complex that it seemed insoluble, I would stop working for a moment, lift my concentrated gaze from the operative field, look up at my assembled team with what I hoped was a mischievous bit of twinkle in my eye, and act like I was tongue-in-cheek kidding when I said, "Do you suppose we'll ever get out of this?" It was a subterfuge that relied on the residents' and nurses' assuming that I would not possibly say such a thing if I really meant it. Their amused responses always lightened the atmosphere, added to the team's solidarity, and allowed me to go back to work with renewed confidence.

Or, of course, there was the other line that always did the trick when I could sense that my assistants or the scrub nurse were becoming overly tense concerning the danger of what was being done, or about some incipient disaster that they be-

lieved might be on the immediate horizon. When their transmitted tension reached the point where I felt it affecting my
calm, I would say, "You know, folks, after I do a case like this
I always send the pants of my scrub suit to the Monarch
Laundry. They don't wash things too well, but they're very
discreet." This seemed to acknowledge to members of the
team that there was justification for their understandable
fear, but that things were so well under control that the surgeon was relaxed enough to make jokes about the situation.

The underlying purpose of all these little bits of subterfuge—none of which, incidentally, were original with
me—was to cut tension and restore the air of equanimity so
necessary for detached thought, without which decision is
impossible and action is paralyzed or worse. Even in the
midst of one's own perturbation, doing something to lessen
the general atmosphere of tension has the effect of blowing
away, at least in part, the incipient panic that inhibits rational
thought. Panic is contagious, but so is a calming influence.

I have been writing here of acute problems, but the same
sort of thinking applies to any long-standing situation in which
the level of stress is such that it threatens the detachment so essential to judgment and wisdom. The mere acknowledgment
of the unavoidable nature of the anxiety inherent in certain
circumstances removes the self-condemnation that may com-
plicate it, and makes matters more relaxed for all concerned.
Taking away blame and granting oneself permission to be less
than imperturbable may be the best path toward the very imperturbability we seek.

Like several of the other characteristics of wisdom, equanimity appears to become easier with age. Studies of large
numbers of the elderly indicate, assuming mental health, that

effective regulation of emotional response is more likely to be found in older men and women than in younger. They are less prone to anger, impatience, bitterness, and negativity than their sons and daughters, and are accordingly able to approach problems with a more balanced attitude. Not only that, but when such undesired moods do appear, they are better managed by older individuals. The restraint that characterizes maturity of mind grows with maturity of years.

Aging can be a process of learning to filter, of choosing to avoid or remove those aspects of response that the years have shown to be counterproductive or even harmful. "The Aristotelian sage," wrote Montaigne, "is not exempt from the emotions: he moderates them." As we grow older, it seems to become less important, for example, to assert the rightness of every position we take, or to express displeasure with every person whose opinions or character do not suit our fancy or measure up to our expectations. "One of the first essentials in securing a good-natured equanimity," wrote Osler, "is not to expect too much of the people amongst whom you dwell. 'Knowledge comes, but wisdom lingers.' " When impatience is less, so is the frustration that leads so quickly to anger. Anger especially has been found to be less frequent, less explosive, and less sustained among the elderly. "The growth of wisdom," wrote Nietzsche, "may be gauged exactly by the diminution of ill temper." Ill temper, aggressiveness, the driving need to win at all costs—they man the barricades against wisdom, and stiffen the resistance to the judicious persuasion so necessary if good judgment is to win the day.

Though nothing can be more important to good judgment than equanimity, equanimity is not the same as being placid, a condition against which older men and women must be on guard. Though few would not admire Miriam Gabler, for example, for the contentment that has been the reward of her later years, contentment can, inappropriately applied, be the enemy of wisdom. Complete peace of mind does not exist, nor would we want it to, especially as it sometimes slides dangerously close to passivity. Wisdom needs a measure of constructive discontent.

The motivating power of discontent is the subject of a chapter in *Man Is Not Alone,* the most highly acclaimed of the religio-philosophical books of the eminent theologian Rabbi Abraham Joshua Heschel. Heschel writes of the importance of a chronic state of dissatisfaction of a particular sort: Man, he proclaims, must "be content with what he *has,* but never with what he *is.*" (Italics in the original.)

> Self-satisfaction, self-fulfillment is a myth which panting souls must find degrading. All that is creative stems from a seed of endless discontent. It is because of men's dissatisfaction with the customs, sanctions and modes of behavior of their age and race that moral progress is possible. New insight begins when satisfaction comes to an end.

In no aspect of wisdom is restraint more necessary than in the manifestation and uses of discontent. Unrestrained discontent can be querulous and quarrelsome, and bears the danger of falling into self-righteousness, another of the enemies of wisdom. The wise travel along the golden mean; they are restrained by caveats of humility spread out like so many signposts along the lengthy road to their goal. "Thus said the

Lord," proclaimed Jeremiah, "Let not the wise man glory in his wisdom."

To be smugly self-righteous is to be rigid, resistant to the openness so crucial to the ongoing search for wisdom, in which so much humility is needed. But openness to change comes with its own caveat: the danger of the impermanent. The capacity to deal with change is the capacity as well to distinguish between the transitory and the steadily evolving culture of a society, an advantage that accrues to age, which has seen so much. Older men and women know that most changes are of the moment. The wise are sensitive to the difference between the ephemeral and the enduring, and seek clues to help them distinguish between the two.

The restraint of the wise keeps them grounded when others are jumping too early onto flashy bandwagons. At the same time, a wise person's openness to change allows a willingness to give up old ways even before they become superannuated. The most quoted poet in the English language chose precisely this subject for one of his most quoted couplets. Alexander Pope wrote in two-lined aphorisms for those who would get wisdom.

> Be not the first by whom the new are tried,
> Nor yet the last to lay the old aside.

And true wisdom lies also in allowing for context. Though wisdom has about it a necessary timelessness, it must also be a thing of its time, place, atmosphere, and circumstances. And here we return to the notion of adaptability. What is wise in one situation may be folly in another. The wise man has traditionally been thought of as a rock of solid dependability, but he is only dependable and his judgment is solid only insofar as his thought is supple.

None of us is born with the inherent gift of wisdom. "Wisdom is the principal thing," we are told in the Book of Proverbs, "therefore get wisdom." But how are we to get it? The question was addressed by Marcel Proust: "We do not receive wisdom; we must discover it for ourselves after a long journey that no one can take for us or spare us." And so, it may again be asked, "But how are we to discover it?" How does a man or woman come to the knowledge, the equanimity, the restraint, the detachment, the *caritas,* the fairness, the foresight, and all those other qualities without which there is no wisdom?

The very fact of wisdom's incompleteness catalyzes the motivation to further the pursuit, as Heschel would certainly advise us. Knowing that an undertaking can never be completed is no reason to turn away from it. The Talmudic sage Rabbi Tarphon is known for having admonished anyone who would hesitate to take on an obligation that by its very nature is impossible to completely fulfill. His oft-quoted exhortation is recorded in the "Pirke Avoth": "The day is short and the work is great, and the laborers are sluggish, and the wages are abundant, and the master of the house is demanding. It is not necessary that you complete the work, but neither are you free to desist from it."

Though we are not free to desist from the hard work of pursuing wisdom, we should never allow ourselves to forget that the wages are abundant—the reward is great. That the process takes more time than is granted by the human life span cannot be doubted, but here the advantages—and the obligations—are all with those who are older. To be wise, one has to have lived, though it must be acknowledged that some men and women, even when young, extract a lot more living from their years than do others.

But wisdom increases with age only for those who never lose their receptiveness to change, and to progress within themselves. For this, an inquiring mind is needed, along with the necessary humility and the conviction that one can never know enough. Wisdom demands unending skepticism, the constant questioning of one's own assumptions and conclusions, and the determination to become better than we are, until the day of our death.

Equanimity is wisdom, *caritas* is wisdom, beneficence is wisdom, and so are all those other qualities so crucial to wisdom's existence. Each of them can be found—can be strengthened, too—at any stage of life. But the long habit of living can make them stronger still. For each of them there is a caveat, a warning against its own overabundance; for the aggregate there is a balance, which in general terms is the balance between expansiveness and restraint. It is for such reasons that the ancient Greeks spoke of the golden mean, and this too is wisdom.

Wisdom means having a certain steadiness of ongoing personal philosophy that is consistent while it is open to change; it means insisting on the primacy of reliable knowledge and truth, while aware that all knowledge should be questioned because there is no absolute truth; being skeptical always, while never cynical; having a justifiable confidence in one's own knowledge and judgment, while granting that they are far from perfect; knowing oneself, while conceding the bias and insecurities that may distort such insight; relying on conscious and unconscious modeling after those whom we believe to be wise, while recognizing that everyone is fallible; feeling a sense of personal involvement and *caritas* for others, while retaining sufficient detachment to aid in fairness and objectivity; transcending one's own needs, while using perception of those needs as a prism through which to see the world; being reflective, while committed to decision and action; being idealistic, while remaining grounded in what is; building peace of mind, while being sufficiently discontented to fuel the engines of necessary reform; anticipating the consequences of one's choices and actions, while conceding the uncertainty of such predictions; accepting cultural change, while being aware of the kind of change that is only ephemeral; thinking timelessly, while being of the time; taking account of the values of one's society and era, while not allowing oneself to be restricted by them; appealing to the best in others while not expecting more of them than they are capable of giving; maintaining a vision of a better tomorrow, while living in the reality of today.

And even with all of it, there is no wisdom without humility. Humility assures that there is never wisdom enough, assures Heschel's "seed of endless discontent," assures that wisdom's pursuit never slackens or ceases. Perhaps because he had so much less of it within himself than he might have wished for, T. S. Eliot expressed his conviction of humility's primacy in his memorable "East Coker":

> *The only wisdom we can hope to acquire*
> *Is the wisdom of humility: humility is endless.*

And there is no wisdom, either, without the constant reevaluation of ourselves—the constant rethinking on all that we have been, all that we are, and all that we can be, regardless of age. Absent that, absent wisdom. Not surprisingly, it is Plato who has the last word, reminding us once more that "the unexamined life is not worth living." A long life of not hesitating to look inward is the key to understanding all that can be seen when we look outward.

TEN

A CODA FOR AGING

*I want Death to find me planting my cabbages, nei-
ther worrying about it nor about the unfinished gar-
dening.*

—Michel de Montaigne, *Essays: To Philosophize
Is to Learn How to Die*, 1580

There is no fountain of youth, but we have nourishing
water fonts of a different sort, much better and more
realistic. These others are the wellsprings all along the
course of our lives, to enrich the flowing current that gradually grows into the fullness of age. Like the moving water itself, our aging is a continuity with everything we have become
since a much earlier stage—everything that has entered the
slowly maturing stream of our being. Self-assurance, optimism, productivity, attachments of *caritas* to others, pride in

our physical selves—these are all philosophies that enhance living. They are wellsprings largely of our own making, and they can grow in significance as we let their energies pour into the ever-widening, deepening channel of experience and wisdom.

Because such qualities become increasingly consequential as the decades pass, we need to begin in youth consciously to think about them, and seek ways to encourage the sources from which they feed the ongoing stream. Even when the flowings that have come together to form our lives are not all we might have wished them to be—whether because of heredity, upbringing, illness, or circumstance—we can knowingly seek the new ones that are to be found along the way, and dig deeply into their sources so that their refreshing influx brings with it the ongoing progress we need if we are to continue being carried forward.

It is never too late to find new tributaries that add vibrancy to our lives. Though the work of finding these sources may be difficult and slow at first, we should not abandon it. The rewards for persistence, as Rabbi Tarphon would remind us, are abundant. And they are abundant at any time of life. But as our sixties and seventies approach, we must increasingly take deliberate steps of our own if betterment is the objective, or even constancy. Less and less is there a choice whether to explore for the resources that enhance our years. Late in life, the exploration becomes mandatory.

The harvest of such explorations can be astonishing, and unpredictable to those of us who were convinced in our middle years that we had already found every avenue to which our interests might take us. Of the rewards of aging, few are more gratifying than the unexpected discoveries we make about ourselves. When Henry Wadsworth Longfellow returned to Bowdoin College for the fiftieth anniversary of his commencement, he brought with him a poem written for his 1825 classmates, *"Morituri Salutamus,"* whose final lines express as well as I have ever encountered the quiet confidence of those who never stop looking for the wellsprings that may appear late in life.

> For age is opportunity no less
> Than youth itself, though in another dress,
> And as the evening twilight fades away
> The sky is filled with stars, invisible by day.

I have now, in the second half of my seventies, spent countless hours knowingly and unknowingly observing older men and women, and myself as well, under conditions ranging from extreme stress—as in life-threatening illness—to extreme tranquility—as in the reassuring warmth of home and family. As a result, I have become convinced that, beyond the pursuit of wisdom, there is a triad of factors that, among others of lesser but nevertheless significant consequence, are the essential ingredients of the benisons that should come with the later decades of our lives. Better that we discover them in youth, but there is no time beyond which they may not bring a flow of renewal to the journey. The three are: a sense of mutual caring and connectedness with others; the maintenance, insofar as we can influence it by our own actions, of the physical capability of our bodies; and creativity. Each of the three requires work; each of the three brings immense rewards.

Though the concept of creativity has not been directly addressed in these pages, it is interwoven into virtually every-

thing that has been said. Think only of the creativity that has
filled the days of some of the men and women encountered
here, a creativity that has taken different forms for each of
them. Sometimes the form of creativity has been on a continuum with all that came before, and sometimes creativity
has made its entry in the form of something entirely new—
whether a wellspring that appeared of its own, or one that required exploration, discovery, and digging to gain access to
its vein of origin.

René La Forestrie is a man who has brought creativity
into the drab existence of men and women in a place one
might assume to be the unlikeliest of locations for such things:
a public home for the aged. La Forestrie's experience as a psy-
chologist of vast experience with an elderly population has
demonstrated that creativity is the key to the vibrancy that
can rekindle the flame of older lives, and bring rewards previously unimagined.

When I met him in 1994, La Forestrie was director of psy-
chology at Charles Foix hospital, a two-thousand-bed state-
supported institution for the aged, located in Ivry-sur-Seine, a
suburb of Paris. As a result of his own long-standing observations, he was certain that some degree of creativity is inherent
in everyone, and so he determined to establish an atmosphere
at Charles Foix that might encourage it in the institutionalized old, a group traditionally so infantilized by society and
caregivers that the probability of achieving such a goal would
seem to be remote. His premise was not only that creativity is
not lost among the elderly, but that men and women in this
age group often have far more to say than does youth, and
are capable of expressing themselves through the medium of
graphic art, even if they had not previously had any experi-

ence with it. With this as a given, he introduced a program that, in fact, is an example of creativity.

The program's aim was to find and set free that inherent creativity. La Forestrie's intent was to let loose a wellspring that had been submerged during youth and middle age by the ordinariness or busyness of his patients' lives, and more recently by their own and others' negativistic attitudes about the aged. Because Charles Foix hospital is a public institution, the backgrounds of its occupants range from the uneducated to men and women with doctorates. It was La Forestrie's contention that such people needed an outlet in order to say what they had to say, in spite of having had no previous idea that they wanted to say anything at all.

He began by inviting a group of Parisian painters—of whom there is no dearth in that most aesthetically attuned of cities—to work pro bono with any patient who wanted to avail him- or herself of the program. Enough ateliers, or studios, were converted from other uses so that all takers among the institution's population might be accommodated. The response was gratifying, especially as so few of the responders had ever studied art before. Each of them was given a key to the atelier in which he or she painted, so that the room might be entered at any time of day or night. Working one-on-one with their aged acolytes, the professional artists found that they could bring out in them inclinations, emotions, and sometimes talents the elderly had never known existed. Most important, the urge to creativity was, in fact, recognized in virtually everyone, less to the astonishment of the instructors and La Forestrie himself than to the men and women discovering this new excitement within themselves.

At the time of my 1994 visit, the program had been going

on for about fifteen years. Standing in one of the ateliers with La Forestrie one overcast wintry afternoon, I found myself gazing figuratively openmouthed at several dozen of the thousands of paintings housed in the institution's collection. Nearby, a blue-kerchiefed woman of perhaps eighty was working quietly and with intense concentration on her latest oeuvre, so deeply immersed in the mixing of her colors that she seemed oblivious to our hushed conversation no more than ten feet from her. Though some of the pictures being shown to me were obviously the work of people who had discovered unsuspected talent, most were not. But each of those in the rather large group of canvases astonished me in its own way, with its expressiveness, its colors and forms, and its meaning to me as an observer. With few exceptions, there seemed evident such a depth of feeling and an artistry of emotion that I have not to this day forgotten the effect that the experience of seeing them had on me.

La Forestrie calls the years of being old *l'âge de créer,* "the age of creating." But he might just as well put the expression backward, and say "the creativity of age." In his program, as he states it so clearly, the perspective of the artist has enabled a liberation in the perspective of the elderly, has enabled an autonomy, has enabled an independence. These newly developed painters have done it, he points out, without self-regard or vanity. Their encounters with creativity have brought about not only a liberation of something powerful and new within them, but a transformation in their aging.

The wellsprings of creativity lie everywhere to be discovered. They may appear in the most improbable of forms and at the most unexpected of times. We should not wait for that appearance—we should actively seek it out, and then attend to the wellspring as if our lives depended on it—which they do, in fact. We must take up every promising opportunity with a sense of purpose, and throw ourselves wholeheartedly into it. For nothing less will bring the satisfaction that comes from allowing ourselves to become so totally immersed in a project that we lose all sense of anything but its importance to us at that moment.

"At that moment." We live in moments, hours, and individual days. This is how things get done. Though the future must be planned for, and though all that we are at any instant is the result of all that we have been in the past, the actual living of our lives occurs in what William Osler a century ago called "day-tight compartments." Addressing an assemblage of Yale students in 1913, he quoted Carlyle, who wrote, "Our main business is not to see what lies dimly at a distance, but to do what lies clearly at hand." At any age, we must engage actively with the present. Be sure to climb a mountain from time to time, he urged, so that you may partake of the wisdom that comes of looking in all directions. Plan for future hopes, but to reach that time lying ahead, we must focus on the work of today: "Absorption in the duty of the hour is in itself the best guarantee of ultimate success." A man may hold a single day in his hand, Osler advised, and in this way make it his own. "The future is to-day," he proclaimed. "The day of a man's salvation is *now*—the life of the present, of to-day, lived earnestly, intently, without a forward-looking thought, is the only insurance for the future. Let the limit of your horizon be a twenty-four hour circle."

Osler understood that commitment brings focus, and only with focus and commitment can come the satisfaction that is the fruit of creativity. When we throw ourselves with intensity and purposefulness into achieving a goal, no matter its nature, the energy applied to the task is directly proportional to the energy generated in us by the creativity in which we justifiably take pride. Pride is a form of energy, and it is fueled by creating something. These things are made possible by the kind of determined concentration on the task at hand, which brings the joy of accomplishment. It is not so much the *what* of what we do, but the dignity, grace, and determination with which we do it. We need accomplishment at any age, but after the hurly-burly of getting and spending has ended and the latter decades approach, it becomes an essential in our sense of self. We do it best by living in day-tight compartments, and immersing ourselves in the now. When William Osler published his address as an essay, he gave it a title that declared it to be his personal philosophy: "A Way of Life."

What we actually do occurs one day at a time. But its choice and its ultimate purpose is part of the panorama of our lives, which we can see only by ascending to that mountaintop often enough to maintain a focus on all that we have been, all that we are, and all that we wish to be. But too much time breathing the thin air on the peak induces vertigo and feelings of unreality, while depriving the climber of the oxygen necessary to get safely down to the plain below, where the real work is done. Still, the expansive view is necessary if we are to use the past and present to plan for the future, and make sure that all the day-tight compartments are well used, and all the synapses well lubricated with neurotransmitters.

What I am getting at with all of these high-altitude metaphors is simply that it is necessary to plan ahead, if old age is to be productive and rewarding. Every stage of life is preparation for the next, and even those beyond. And yet, we do so little to get ready for our own aging, other than to assure a financial nest egg and perhaps buy long-term-care insurance. In fact, some mistakenly believe that retirement is the time to abandon everything that has come before, as if that were possible. They escape to a sun belt of expectations that too often leaves them dissatisfied and seeking ways to relieve the ennui.

Old age must be based on a foundation built during the decades that precede it; it is not enough to do the best we can when the years have already overtaken us. Beginning in middle age, we must study how to be old, in somewhat the same way that we, when growing up, studied to be adults, and prepared for the coming responsibilities by educating our minds and strengthening our bodies. In its own way, aging is an art form—in itself a type of creativity.

The later years require wisdom even more than do the decades that have preceded them. Like the earlier ones, the later years must be approached with the conviction that they can be creative, and can contribute to the well-being of others. The wisdom—and the art, too—consists of understanding, preparing, and making the adjustments that will bring about such a portrait of age, and burnish it to an image of grace and goodness. The changes that gradually occur in our bodies must be perceived for what they are: messages that the wise have taught themselves to interpret in such a way that the best may yet be taken from every day, and every opportunity. Like all art, such a consummation demands vigilance, forethought, and application, and all of these can bring immense pleasure and the satisfaction that comes with the success of achievement.

The majority of readers of this book will live beyond their eightieth year, and some far beyond. If no preparations have been made for that probability—no serious thought given to it—now is the time to begin. I do not mean by this the practical preparations such as the financial or even the thorough health evaluation without which no man or woman should reach late middle age. What I mean is the cultivation of a worldview, an outlook with which to welcome rather than merely face the years and perhaps decades ahead—a way of life, to apply Osler's words in a somewhat different context. If it is true, as Robert Butler, among the wisest of our seers of aging, puts it, that the baby boomers will be a "transformational generation . . . helping to transform old age," then each boomer bears the responsibility to stand for periods of time on the top of the mountain, to look in every direction, and then to act—for his or her own sake and for the sake of those who come after them.

This book has not been about eating granola and emulating Okinawans, although there can be no doubt that these are good things to do; this book is about mind and spirit. We do, after all, put away money in a pension fund for our old age. Why not also prepare ourselves emotionally by putting away spiritual and intellectual capital? Why not prepare ourselves physically, by becoming accustomed to regular vigorous exercise and proper diet long before they become crucial to avoiding frailty? Why not prepare ourselves with a cultivation of the *caritas* that can bring untold rewards to every stage of our lives? Like a well-run pension fund, what we put in is proportional to what we get out, and the interest keeps growing.

And why not, earlier than we might have thought, begin to separate ourselves from the certainty that our career is our identity? Though we may define ourselves primarily by the occupation we have chosen for our life's work, it cannot be allowed to be the only mirror in which we are reflected. Ideally, the balance has been there from the beginning, but hardly always. As the middle years slip imperceptibly into the later, our total humanity—always at the true basis of what we are—must be allowed to emerge as the guiding force of our lives, the total humanity that allows the full expression of *caritas*. These are things for which we prepare by letting them rise gradually to the surface, long before our careers in the marketplace have begun to dwindle, or have come to an abrupt halt.

It has been my observation that in the first forty or fifty years of our lives, we devote much thought and industry to being like others, emulating those we admire, and fitting into a mold that enables us to fill the desired and admired niche in the trajectory of a career and a social station. When not influenced by the vanity and false values so often surrounding us, much of this is to the good, because it is the pathway to understanding the ambience in which we live, and a pattern for worldly success. Not only that, but this is how we gather the knowledge and experience so crucial to the getting of wisdom. During all of this time, we are consciously and unconsciously discovering which parts of that accumulated observation fit best into our own system of values, and we are absorbing these parts into ourselves. So long as we are actively engaged in career, we must abide more or less strictly to the boundaries imposed by it. But once we begin to separate ourselves, we bit by bit become freer to continue maturing in ways distinctive to ourselves.

By such means, age becomes a liberator. All that we have absorbed in a lifetime of attention to others and the world around us becomes the wherewithal for the uniqueness that can now reach the zenith of its fulfillment. The better we have used our years, the greater will be the rewards of individuality and accrued wisdom. As Leonardo da Vinci wrote in the *Codex Atlanticus,* "If you are mindful that old age has wisdom for its food, you will so exert yourself in youth, that your old age will not lack sustenance."

ACKNOWLEDGMENTS

Always absent from a book's Acknowledgments section is the unacknowledged convention that the name of spouse, lover, or best friend (or all three when they are embodied in the same person, as they are in this case) must always be saved for the very end, as though the climax of a crescendo built up by the preceding paragraphs.

I am married to a very impatient woman. Though not given to discouragement, wavering, or loss of will when matters are great, she chafes at delay when matters are small, as in restaurants, traffic jams, and the inanimate automation of telephone trees. Since it is in my power in this one instance to put her before everyone else, I will turn convention on its head by following the lead described in the Gospel of St. Matthew, by which "Many that are first shall be last; and the last shall be first." This last is the very least I owe to the most perceptive editor I have ever had, whether of my writing or my life. If my thesis in describing moral imagination is correct—and I am certain that it is—I am a far better man for the long habit of looking into her eyes and seeing myself reflected there. And if it is also true that wisdom grows with the strength of certain relationships of *caritas*—and I am certain that it does—I can lay claim for this single reason if for no other to being the wisest of men. This book owes any clarity it may have to Sarah Peterson's uncompromising intelligence.

And it owes so much as well, to my editor, Robert Loomis. For years, I have nourished the hope that circumstances might one day be such that Bob and I would work on a book together, and it has finally happened. As rewarding as my fantasy had predicted our collaboration would be, the reality has exceeded even the high expectation. He has guided this book in ways obvious and subtle, and given me the honor I now claim, which is to call him my friend.

And as for friendships, Glen Hartley began ours with a phone call out of the blue, late on a Thursday afternoon some fifteen years ago. He and Lynn Chu have been the staunchest of advocates and the most determined of literary agents. To be represented by them is to be understood as a writer and to be appreciated as a man trying to articulate a vision of the human experience.

For some thirty-five years, the personal and moral philosophies of Vittorio Ferrero have been my constant guide, and the model on which I have based my view of the world and all it has come to mean. We have been more than friends and even more than brothers. Our patterns of thinking have become interwoven one into the other, though my small gifts to him pale in comparison to all he has given me.

Accelerated in the last few years, this book—like its author—has been in progressive stages of development for three quarters of a century. Some of the ideas and thoughts described here were evolving decades before I had any awareness that they were in the process of formation. So many men and women have contributed to every phase of the evolution, that I can thank only those whom I have sought out during the actual writing. Each of them has been forthcoming, frank, and helpful beyond my ability to describe in the small space of a few allotted pages; each of them has made me look in directions and explore issues I might not have considered without the suggestions they made and the questions they raised.

For me, the voice of my Yale colleague, Leo Cooney, has been the voice of authority and reason, not only in geriatrics and gerontology, but in the entire spectrum of caring for the human body and spirit. He has been generous with his time, his counsel, and his good nature. Our hours together have provided insights that affect every chapter that appears between these covers.

Jason Pontin, first as the editor of *Acumen: Journal of Sciences* and later of MIT's *Technology Review,* suggested that I write the essays later incorporated into chapters 7 and 8. As though intuiting that it was time for me to begin marshaling my voluminous though still scattered notions about aging, he not only put my feet to the fire, but actually thought up a notion that eventually found its way into the subtitle of my book. And so, he has been both a human catalyst and a bit of parent as well, to the finished product.

Books of this kind are virtually impossible to write without the help of a skilled research assistant. I have been blessed with the appearance in my life of a young woman on the brink of her own brilliant academic career, who has been unstinting in her devotion to this project and every other one in which I've been engaged in recent years. Christiana Peppard's instincts, her industry, and her intellect have been instrumental in so many ways as the work progressed that my debt to her is exceeded in magnitude only by the joy it has given me to know her.

Not a single one of those friends whom I approached hesitated for a moment in an enthusiastic willingness to discuss issues of aging, to read and comment on sections or all of the manuscript, or to help guide my thinking into forms that I might articulate to a general reader. Because I admire each of them so much, I am proud to put their names in these pages. They are Cornelia and Michael Bessie, Sam Litzinger, John Mascotte, Dorcas MacClintock, Robert Massey, Patricia Papper, James Ponet, Kathleen Queen Peterson, and Lyn Traverse.

And so, there they are—in a reversal of the usual order. I am grateful for all they have done, but even more so because the writing of this book has brought me closer to each of them.

New Haven, 2007

INDEX

ABOUT THE AUTHOR

SHERWIN B. NULAND is Clinical Professor of Surgery at the Yale School of Medicine. Dr. Nuland is the author of *How We Die,* which won the National Book Award and was a finalist for the Pulitzer Prize and the Book Critics Circle Award, as well as *Lost in America, The Doctors' Plague, Leonardo da Vinci,* and *How We Live.* He lives in Connecticut.

ABOUT THE TYPE

This book was set in Sabon, a typeface designed by the well-known German typographer Jan Tschichold (1902–1974). Sabon's design is based upon the original letter forms of Claude Garamond and was created specifically to be used for three sources: foundry type for hand composition, Linotype, and Monotype. Tschichold named his typeface for the famous Frankfurt typefounder Jacques Sabon, who died in 1580.